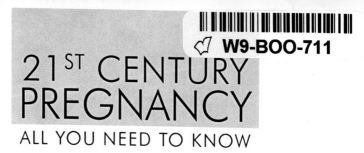

21ST CENTURY
PREGNANCY
ALL YOU NEED TO KNOW

Nine
Healthy
Months

W9-BOO-711

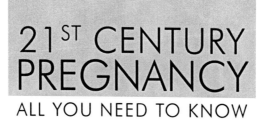

21ST CENTURY PREGNANCY
ALL YOU NEED TO KNOW

Nine Healthy Months

CHARLES HUX, MD
Maternal & Fetal Medicine Specialist

iUniverse, Inc.
New York   Bloomington

Copyright © 2009 by Charles Hux, MD

Interior line drawings © Robert Schoolcraft

Special thanks to Carolyn Tedeschi, cover model and patient.

All rights reserved. No part of this book may be used or reproduced by
any means, graphic, electronic, or mechanical, including photocopying,
recording, taping or by any information storage retrieval system
without the written permission of the publisher except in the case
of brief quotations embodied in critical articles and reviews.
The information, ideas, and suggestions in this book are not
intended as a substitute for professional medical advice.
Before following any suggestions contained in this book, you
should consult your personal physician. Neither the author
nor the publisher shall be liable or responsible for any loss
or damage allegedly arising as a consequence of your use or
application of any information or suggestions in this book.

iUniverse books may be ordered through booksellers or by contacting:

iUniverse
1663 Liberty Drive
Bloomington, IN 47403
www.iuniverse.com
1-800-Authors (1-800-288-4677)

Because of the dynamic nature of the Internet, any Web addresses or links
contained in this book may have changed since publication and may no longer be
valid. The views expressed in this work are solely those of the author and do not
necessarily reflect the views of the publisher, and the publisher hereby disclaims
any responsibility for them.

ISBN: 978-1-4401-3985-7 (sc)
ISBN: 978-1-4401-3988-8 (dj)
ISBN: 978-1-4401-3987-1 (ebook)

Printed in the United States of America

iUniverse rev. date:7/14/2009

Contents

Part 6: Maternal Medical Complications

Part 7: Complications of Pregnancy

Part 8: Things to Consider Before You Deliver

Part 9: Labor, Delivery, and Postpartum

Resource Appendix

Preface

For the past 25 years, I have been counseling my patients on many different topics regarding their pregnancies. I thought it was time to put together a book on the most common questions and concerns my patients have.

There is nothing more exciting than the anticipation of bringing a new life into this world. A natural maternal instinct is to want to do everything in your power to ensure that your baby has the best start in life. I want you to use this book to make sure that you have all the information you need to make that happen.

With so much information out there, many mothers-to-be are not quite sure what is fact and what is fiction. The information in this book has the most up-to-date facts that you'll need in order to make informed choices regarding the well-being of your unborn baby. It will also explain what you need to do for yourself to make sure you stay healthy during and after your pregnancy.

I cover many topics that are not addressed in other pregnancy books. I also let you know what is both common and rare in pregnancy. This is important because some books choose to discuss very rare events in great detail. I have found that many women will then dwell on this very rare event, worrying that their pregnancy will also be affected.

This book lets you read about any topic in five minutes. I did not want to waste your time going into too much detail about information you really don't need. My short summaries give you the important facts on each topic and explain some complicated topics in easy-to-understand language.

I hope this book will answer many of your questions, but it should never be used to replace the advice your doctor gives you.

I hope you find this book useful during your pregnancy, and I hope your pregnancy is a wonderful journey that brings you a very healthy and happy baby.

Charles Hux, MD

Acknowledgments

I wish to extend my sincere thanks to Marla Jensen for her contribution and dedication to this book. I could never have done this without you.

I would also like to thank Dr. Ronald Wapner, my mentor and friend.

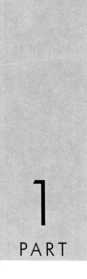

1

PART

PRE-PREGNANCY ISSUES

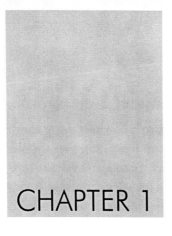

CHAPTER 1

Steps to Take before Getting Pregnant

Whether this is your first or fifth upcoming pregnancy, you should want to be in the best health possible for this new human being you are bringing into the world.

You can take many steps before you get pregnant to ensure a successful pregnancy. These include the following:

1. Make an appointment with your primary care physician.

The very first thing you should do is make an appointment with your primary care physician to have your blood checked for anemia and other common problems. Make certain that your blood pressure is normal and your urine is free of any bacteria. You should also make sure that all your immunizations are up to date and that you do not need any boosters.

If you see specific physicians for a chronic illness, get in touch with those doctors so that they are aware you are going to try to get pregnant soon. You might need to have certain medications that you are taking adjusted or switched. If you know you have a chronic illness that might make your pregnancy problematic, it would be a good idea to schedule a pre-conception consultation with a high-risk specialist that deals with these types of pregnancies.

2. Discontinue use of birth control.

If you take birth control pills or are using another form of hormonal birth control, such as the patch, you should discontinue its use and wait two to three menstrual cycles before you try to conceive. This will allow your menstrual cycle to become regulated. Use of condoms during this time is recommended.

3. Begin taking vitamins.

Start taking a daily vitamin that contains at least 400 mcg of folic acid and vitamin B6 before conceiving.

4. Choose your obstetrical provider.

If you do not already have an obstetrical provider for your future care, it would be best to meet with a few providers to see if you are a good fit with their practice.

5. Take care of any dental needs.

If you have not been to the dentist in a while for a cleaning, it would be best to schedule an appointment and have any necessary dental work performed.

6. Get in the best shape possible.

If you need to lose weight, take a few months to adopt a healthy way of eating. Do not think of it as a diet, but rather a change in the way you eat. Eating healthier as you go into the pregnancy will make it much easier to stay on a good balanced diet during the pregnancy. If you haven't been exercising, it is always best to start a program before you get pregnant.

7. Quit smoking.

If you smoke, do whatever you need to do to stop smoking. Smoking is by far the most dangerous thing you can do to yourself and your unborn child.

8. Know your genetic history.

Check the family history for both you and your partner. It is always best to know beforehand if there are any genetic problems that run in the family.

9. Understand your maternity leave options.

If you work, check your company's policy on maternity leave. You will also want to find out how the Family Medical Leave Act (FMLA) works for you. You can usually get this information from your company's human resource department or in your company's employee manual.

10. Know your health insurance benefits.

You should check with your health insurance company to see if you are covered for maternity benefits or, if yours is a newer policy, if there is a preexisting-condition clause for pregnancy. It is important to find out what exactly your insurance will cover and what they won't. Certain plans only let you see participating providers, so make sure the one you will be using is covered under your plan.

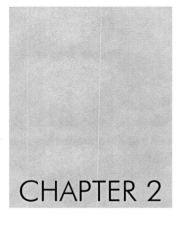

CHAPTER 2

Choosing Your Healthcare Provider

Before you decide on who is going to care for you during your pregnancy, there are many important aspects to consider.

 Be sure to choose a doctor with whom you feel comfortable.

If you already have a gynecologist that you feel comfortable with, who also practices obstetrics, it is probably a good idea to stay with this doctor. However, you may want to consider switching doctors if you are not happy with the hospital where this doctor delivers.

If you are looking for a more natural approach, and your ob/gyn does not have a midwife as part of their practice or your ob/gyn will not work with your birth plan, you may want to seek out a nurse-midwife practice. A nurse-midwife is specially trained in pregnancy and childbirth and will care for you very much the same way as an obstetrician would, but with a more personalized approach. If a problem should occur during your pregnancy, a midwife can always refer you to an obstetrician or high-risk specialist for evaluation.

You may also want to seek out a different doctor if your current ob/gyn does not handle high-risk pregnancies and a chronic medical condition or poor obstetrical history puts your pregnancy in a high-risk category. Maternal-fetal medicine (high-risk) specialists are very much like primary ob/gyns, except they have special training in high-risk pregnancies and medical problems that may complicate a pregnancy. Many also have special training in genetics and detection of birth defects.

 Understand the differences between having a doctor in a solo practice and having a doctor in a group practice.

If you are the type of person that prefers a more one-on-one, close doctor-patient relationship, you might want to consider using a doctor in a solo practice rather than a large group practice where you will see different doctors. However, one important point to consider when picking someone in a solo practice is that they can be called to the hospital to tend to other patients and may not always be able to see you at your scheduled office visit. Also, if your doctor isn't available at the time of delivery, you may have to be delivered by a doctor you have never had the opportunity to meet.

The advantage to using a group practice is that you are assured of an available doctor with whom you already are familiar should you have a problem in the office or the hospital. The main disadvantage of using a group practice is that you may not like all the doctors and won't have control over who will be your delivering physician.

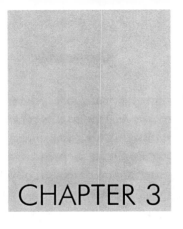

CHAPTER 3

Becoming Pregnant Over the Age of 35

More and more women are becoming pregnant after the age of 35. Even though 35 is still a relatively young age, once you are 35 and pregnant you are defined as being of "advanced maternal age" or AMA.

If you are over 35 and trying to conceive, you should be aware that it might take you a little longer than a younger woman. About one-third of women over the age of 35 will experience fertility problems. The decline in fertility is usually due to less frequent ovulation, diminished egg quality, or endometriosis.

Prenatal care is especially important because older pregnant women are more likely to experience high blood pressure, gestational diabetes, placental problems, and premature delivery. The older you are when you get pregnant will also increase your rate of miscarriage. The miscarriage rate after the age of 35 is about 25 percent.

Babies born to women over 35 have an increased risk of being low birth weight, stillborn, or large for gestational age. Being over 35 also increases your risk of having a child with a chromosome abnormality. This is due to the fact that the quality of a woman's eggs decreases with age. The older you are, the higher the risk becomes. A 35-year-old woman has a 1 in 270 risk of having a baby with a chromosome abnormality; a 40-year-old woman has a 1 in 80 risk, and a 45-year-old woman has a 1 in 30 risk.

Women of advanced maternal age will generally see their doctors more often during the pregnancy. Women over 35 with high-risk factors and all women over 40 should begin weekly antenatal testing at 34 weeks' gestation until delivery. This consists of biophysical profile-testing and Doppler studies to assess the well-being of the baby. As long as the testing is normal, the baby should be fine until your visit the following week.

Most women over 35 can achieve a successful pregnancy. However, if you are overweight, smoke, or already have any chronic medical condition, such as high blood pressure, diabetes, thyroid disease, or heart disease, you should have a consultation with your doctor before you get pregnant to go over these problems.

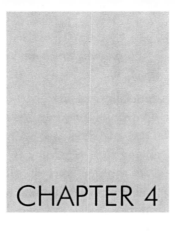

CHAPTER 4

Use of Assisted Reproductive Technology

Infertility is defined as the failure to become pregnant after one year of normal sexual activity without the use of contraception. This occurs in 10–15 percent of all couples.

Many factors can contribute to the infertility of a couple. Female causes of infertility account for about 70 percent of cases. The most common female causes are ovulation dysfunction, anatomical abnormalities of the reproductive system, and endometriosis. Male causes of infertility account for about 30 percent of cases. The most common male cause of infertility is a low sperm count.

Infertility places an incredible stress on a couple, and psychotherapy or counseling is a critical part of the treatment plan for any couple undergoing medical evaluation and treatment for infertility. The basic workup to determine a cause is faster for the man, taking perhaps a couple of weeks. Women's tests can take up to several months before an answer is available.

There are times when a cause is not found, and other times a problem is identified. If a problem is found and treatment still fails to produce a pregnancy, a couple may need to turn to the use of assisted reproductive technology.

This can include the use of infertility drugs, such as Clomid or Pergonal, that stimulate a woman's egg production, as well as *intrauterine insemination* or IUI. IUI is a process that involves the cleaning of a man's sperm and injecting it directly into a woman's uterus at the time of ovulation. It is the safest and most natural method of assisted reproductive technology.

If these methods fail, a couple may turn to the use of *in vitro fertilization* or IVF. This process involves removing a number of eggs from a woman's ovary and then fertilizing them in a laboratory dish with the man's sperm. After several days, the fertilized eggs are then placed back into the woman's uterus in the hope they will implant.

In vitro fertilization (IVF) is frequently used today to achieve successful fertilization and has resulted in thousands of successful pregnancies. However, use of IVF results in a significant increase in preterm births, small (for gestational age) newborns, birth defects and a 20- to 30-fold increase in multiple gestations. Because of the large risk of multiple gestations, the current recommendations are that one to two eggs be placed in women younger than 30, and no more than two to three eggs in women over 30. Some of these higher risks are not due to IVF, but to the fact that women of advanced maternal age who also have chronic medical diseases are getting pregnant when they otherwise would not be able to conceive.

Risks associated with multiple gestations include an increase in preeclampsia, diabetes, preterm delivery, birth defects, and the need for C-sections.

The American College of Obstetrics and Gynecology strongly recommends that all couples undergoing assisted reproductive technologies be counseled on the significant risks of multiple gestations, multi-fetal pregnancy reductions (the need to reduce the number of viable fetuses in the womb), and IVF before undergoing any procedure or using fertility drugs.

Since the mid-1980s, assisted reproductive technology using many new techniques has helped couples with conception. Reproductive endocrinologists have assisted tens of thousands of couples in celebrating the miracle of pregnancy and life, when many would be childless without their help.

Multi-Fetal Pregnancy Reduction

One of the risks of using super ovulation drugs or IVF with multiple-embryo transfer is becoming pregnant with a high-order multiple pregnancy. This is why it is so important to be counseled about the possible risks before undergoing any treatment.

If you become pregnant with three or more fetuses, you may be faced with making a decision about terminating one or more of the fetuses. This option will likely be offered to you by your doctor to improve the chance of survival and reduce the long-term morbidity of the remaining fetuses. You, of course, also have the option to continue the pregnancy with all the fetuses or to terminate the entire pregnancy.

If you choose to undergo fetal reduction, you may wonder how it is determined which baby, or babies, are selected to be reduced. First, it would be suggested that all of the fetuses be tested for any chromosomal abnormalities with the use of CVS or an early amniocentesis. If the testing reveals an abnormality, the affected fetuses would be reduced first. If no abnormalities are detected with any of the fetuses, or if you choose not to have any diagnostic testing performed, the fetuses furthest away from the cervix would be reduced. The optimal time for performing a reduction is in the late-first or early-second trimester. Multi-fetal reduction does carry risks, including total pregnancy loss or loss of one of the remaining fetuses. The risk of a complication from the procedure is between 2 and 4 percent.

Since the ultimate goal of using assisted reproductive technology is to conceive a child, the thought of possibly needing to undergo such a procedure is sure to cause much stress and sadness. If you do choose to reduce a pregnancy, you can expect to grieve the loss just as anyone losing any pregnancy would. Know in the end that you did what you felt you needed to do for yourself and the well-being of your unborn babies.

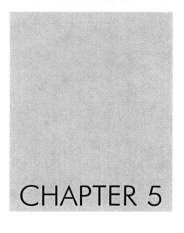

CHAPTER 5

Polycystic Ovarian Syndrome (PCOS)

Polycystic ovarian syndrome (PCOS) is a condition that affects a woman's fertility, hormones, menstrual cycle, insulin production, and circulatory system. If you have been receiving treatment for PCOS, you must inform your ob/gyn, because some of these drugs may not be safe for use during your pregnancy.

Women with PCOS are at an increased risk of developing high blood pressure, preeclampsia, gestational diabetes, and blood-clotting disorders. Pregnant women with PCOS also have a much higher risk of having a miscarriage.

There are steps you can take to reduce your chances of having complications during your pregnancy. If you are overweight, losing some weight will reduce your risk of high blood pressure and miscarriage. Weight loss will also reduce the amount of insulin that your body needs to function.

Most treatments for PCOS are geared toward stabilizing your hormones. This increases your chances of having an uneventful pregnancy.

Your doctor should check your blood pressure at each visit and be on the lookout for early signs of gestational diabetes and preeclampsia toward the end of your pregnancy. Certain medications may also be prescribed to prevent blood clotting.

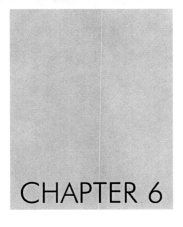

CHAPTER 6

Getting Pregnant While on Birth Control

On occasion, a woman may become pregnant while on oral contraceptives or with an IUD (intrauterine device) in place.

The chance of becoming pregnant when taking oral contraceptives is stated to be about 1 percent, or 1 in 100 women will become pregnant over the course of a year. There are no significant risks to the unborn child's exposure to today's low-hormone oral contraceptives. If you discover that you are pregnant, you should stop use of the pill and contact your doctor.

If you become pregnant and have an IUD in place, see your obstetrician/gynecologist as soon as possible. The chance of getting pregnant with an IUD in place is about 0.5 percent. There are two options if you become pregnant with an IUD in place. You can either have the IUD removed by your doctor or leave it in place throughout the pregnancy. A decision about removal depends on how far along you are into the pregnancy. Removal very early (less than 10 weeks) is the usual plan, which presents a very low risk of pregnancy loss. Leaving the IUD in the uterus increases the risk for preterm delivery and premature rupture of membranes.

All options should be discussed with your doctor.

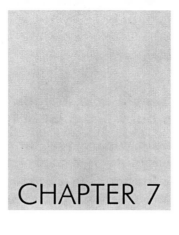

CHAPTER 7

Common Myths about Pregnancy

Is my baby in danger if the umbilical cord is near or around the neck?

This is by far the most commonly asked question by all expectant mothers during any visit to my office. The cord is around the neck or another part of the body in up to half of all fetuses near term. The chance of a cord being wrapped around a part of the baby and causing injury is extremely small (less than one in 2,000 pregnancies). However, during labor, a tightly wrapped cord or a cord tied in a knot may result in the delivery being performed by C-section.

Is dental work, including dental x-rays, done during the pregnancy dangerous for the fetus?

Dental work, x-rays, local anesthesia, and antibiotics are all fine during your pregnancy and do not pose any serious risk to the fetus.

Can reaching up to get something or raising my hands above my head strangle my baby in the womb?

No, that is just not true, but I hear this concern from patients all the time.

❓ If I have severe acid indigestion, does that mean the baby has a lot of hair?

That might be wishful thinking, but the answer is no. Acid indigestion during pregnancy is due to hormones that relax the muscles in your digestive tract. This allows stomach acids to move back up into the esophagus causing a burning sensation.

❓ If I drank a little alcohol before I knew I was pregnant, will that hurt or deform my baby?

The answer is no.

❓ If I am carrying low, does that mean the baby may be ready to deliver?

No, it just means that your uterus tilts forward, which can happen with some pregnancies.

❓ Can having sex cause me to go into premature labor and deliver early?

There is no evidence that having sex contributes to an increase in preterm birth, unless you have a previous preterm birth history or are at risk in this pregnancy. In a "normal" pregnancy, it is common for you to feel a few contractions after having sex, but that does not increase your risk for going into preterm labor or delivering early.

❓ Is it true that if the baby's heartbeat is slow, it's a boy, and if it's fast, it's a girl?

Well that's true about half of the time. The answer is that the fetal heart rate varies between 120 and 160 beats per minute and is faster in the first and early second trimester. The average heart rate is very similar for males and females and cannot be used to determine the sex.

❓ Is it true that you should not take baths while pregnant?

If you are having a normal, uncomplicated pregnancy, it is fine to take baths. If you have had a *cerclage* (a stitch in the cervix) placed for cervical incompetence, you should not take baths.

❓ Is it safe to be near a room that is being painted?

Paint fumes do not have any association with causing fetal birth defects. If you have allergies or asthma, just make sure the room is well ventilated.

❓ Is it true that you should not stand in front of a microwave when it is on or sit in front of a computer terminal?

This is not true. Modern microwave ovens and computer terminals do not expose the baby to harmful radiation.

❓ Will spicy food trigger labor?

This is not true, but it might trigger some indigestion.

❓ If you do not experience morning sickness, does this mean you do not have a strong pregnancy?

This is not true. Many women feel perfectly fine throughout their first trimester and have totally normal, healthy pregnancies.

❓ Is it true that an amniocentesis is performed through a woman's belly button?

This is not the case. It is performed at the best location on the abdomen to access the amniotic fluid.

? Is it true that you should not eat nuts during your pregnancy because the baby might then have a nut allergy?

Currently, there is no scientific proof that avoiding highly allergenic food like nuts during pregnancy will prevent allergies in infants.

? If I am carrying small, does that mean I am having a small baby?

It certainly can mean that the baby is smaller than average; however, most women who look small simply have ligaments that hold the uterus deeper inside the abdomen, and the baby is of normal size.

? Is it true that it is safe to use a fetal Doppler at home to listen to the baby's heartbeat?

It is perfectly safe to occasionally listen to the baby's heartbeat; however, some studies have shown that it can be damaging to the inner ear of the fetus if the Doppler is used on a daily basis.

? Is it true that it is not safe to color your hair when you are pregnant?

While there is a theoretical risk, studies have not come up with anything conclusive to show a cause-and-effect relationship. If you are really concerned, you should wait till the end of the first trimester before you go for that touch-up.

? Do fetal hiccups indicate a problem with the baby?

Fetal hiccups are completely normal during pregnancy and should not be a cause of concern.

2
PART

YOUR CHANGING BODY

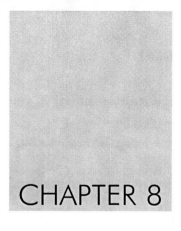

CHAPTER 8

Your Changing Body through Pregnancy

Some women experience many signs and symptoms of pregnancy, while others hardly know they are pregnant. If any of the symptoms that have been listed interfere with your daily life or become severe, you should notify your doctor immediately.

Below is a list of common symptoms you may experience during your pregnancy:

 The First Trimester (Week 1–Week 12)

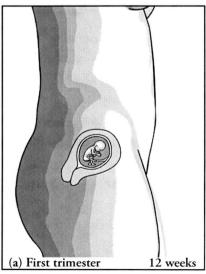

(a) First trimester   12 weeks

o   You may experience nausea and vomiting.

o   You may feel more tired.

o   You may experience heartburn and acid indigestion.

o   You may have to urinate more often.

o   You may become more sensitive to smell.

o   You may have a darkening of the area around the nipple (areola).

o   You may experience sensitivity in your gums and possibly bleeding gums.

o   You may experience increased saliva, with a metallic taste.

o   Your breasts may be swollen and tender.

o   You may crave certain foods.

o   You may have headaches.

o   You may experience mood swings.

o   You may become constipated.

o   You may experience some light spotting.

o   You may have an increase in vaginal discharge.

o   You may experience increased perspiration.

o   You may experience dizziness.

o   You may break out with acne.

o   You may notice that your nails and hair are healthier and growing faster.

 ## The Second Trimester (Week 13–Week 26)

o   You may still be experiencing heartburn and acid indigestion.

o   Your extremities may start to swell from extra fluid.

o   You may experience increased hunger now that your hormones have leveled out.

o   Your breasts may start to increase in size.

o   You may have nasal congestion and nosebleeds.

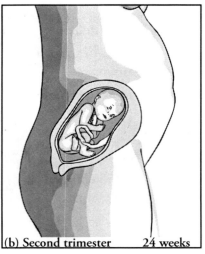

(b) Second trimester   24 weeks

- You may feel achy in your lower abdomen from stretching ligaments.
- Your abdomen may feel itchy from your expanding belly.
- You may notice varicose veins on your legs that can be painful.
- You heart rate may increase.
- Your legs and back may begin to ache.
- A dark line (linea nigra) that runs from your belly button to the pubic bone may appear.
- You may experience pigment changes (chloasma) on your face and neck.
- You should be gaining weight.
- You may feel your baby move between 18 and 22 weeks.

The Third Trimester (Week 27–Week 40)

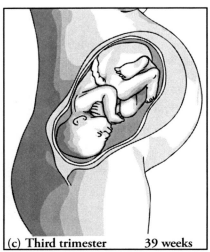

(c) Third trimester   39 weeks

- You may have frequent urination from the baby pressing on your bladder.
- Your weight should continue to increase.
- You may have rib pain from the baby stretching out.
- You may experience hemorrhoids.
- Your belly button may protrude.
- Your saliva may begin to increase again.

- You may have shortness of breath from the baby pressing on your diaphragm.
- You may start to experience painless uterine contractions (Braxton Hicks).
- You may experience a watery discharge (colostrum) leaking from your breasts.
- You may start to notice stretch marks on your abdomen, breasts, and arms.
- You may experience backaches, along with continued leg aches.
- Swelling of your extremities may get worse this trimester.
- You may experience a heavy vaginal discharge.
- You may get itchy red bumps on your belly (PUPP rash).
- You may have alternating periods of fatigue and bursts of energy.

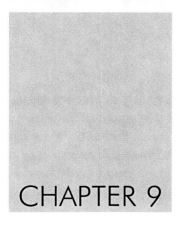

CHAPTER 9

Morning Sickness

Nausea and vomiting in pregnancy, jointly known as "morning sickness," affect approximately 80 percent of all pregnant women. Morning sickness usually begins around the sixth week of pregnancy. Although common in the morning, it can happen almost any time of the day. The majority of women will start feeling much better by the 12th week of pregnancy. Some women will continue to suffer for longer than 12 weeks, and some of these will feel its effects for the duration of their pregnancy.

About 1 percent of pregnant women will experience excessive nausea and vomiting (hyperemesis gravidarum). This condition can cause weight loss, dehydration, and electrolyte imbalance. It is usually treated with Reglan, Zofran, or Phenergan, all Class B medications that are safe if needed in pregnancy. In some cases, hyperemesis gravidarum is so severe that hospitalization is required. Intravenous fluids are usually administered to restore hydration, electrolytes, vitamins, and nutrients.

If the above medications are not working in pill form and you would prefer not to be admitted to the hospital, the use of Reglan and Zofran can be administered at home through a micro-infusion pump. Receiving these medications in this manner can be more effective in certain patients that do not get relief from using these drugs in pill form.

The exact cause of nausea and vomiting in pregnancy remains

unknown. The most widely accepted reason is from the buildup of hCG (human chorionic gonadotropin) in your body. This is the hormone produced after the embryo implants, which will level off by the second trimester. Estrogen is another hormone that rises rapidly in pregnancy and could play a role. Some women may have an underlying gastric condition, such as gallstones or small bowel disease, that is exacerbated when pregnant.

Whatever the reason, morning sickness isn't harmful to your pregnancy but can be quite an uncomfortable side effect of it.

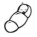 ## Steps to try to make the experience more manageable:

- Eat small, frequent meals during the day so that your stomach is never empty.
- Avoid fatty foods, which are harder to digest.
- Stay away from spicy, fried foods and acidic foods that can irritate your stomach.
- Do not lie down right after a meal. Give yourself some time to digest.
- Munch on crackers throughout the day.
- Eat starchy foods, such as pasta, rice, or potatoes.
- Take your prenatal vitamin with food.
- Ginger—this remedy is thought to help settle your stomach and ease nausea.
- Try acupuncture bands or the Relief Wrist Band.
- Take 100 mg of vitamin B6 each day.
- Be sure to rest or nap during the day.

You should always try non-medicinal remedies first. If nothing you have tried has worked, talk with your healthcare provider about over-the-counter remedies and medications that can be prescribed.

CHAPTER 10

What Do Those hCG Levels Mean?

Human chorionic gonadotropin (hCG) is a hormone produced by the placenta at the moment implantation first takes place. When you buy a home pregnancy test, this is the hormone being measured in your urine. If there is any hCG hormone in your body, then you are very likely pregnant. The hCG is detectable even before you miss your period with the new, highly sensitive tests now available in drug stores. A home pregnancy test does not give you a level of hCG hormone, it will just indicate whether it's present or not.

A doctor will not routinely measure your hCG levels unless some type of problem is encountered, such as early bleeding or cramping. However, if an early transvaginal ultrasound performed between five and eight weeks' gestation cannot identify a viable fetus, you will be sent for quantitative hCG testing. This testing involves having your blood drawn and then having it drawn again three days later.

Detectable levels of hCG start at 5 mIU/ml during the first week of gestation. In a healthy pregnancy, blood levels of hCG will double every 36 hours. There is a great variation in hCG levels. The level itself doesn't matter as much as the rate of change in the level. So if your doctor reports a low number after your first quantitative hCG, do not be discouraged. As long as the number doubles, this would indicate a viable pregnancy. Falling hCG levels always indicate a non-viable pregnancy.

3
PART

BABY'S DEVELOPMENT

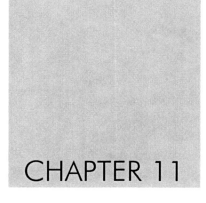

CHAPTER 11

Your Baby's Development Month by Month

 ### Month 1

Conception typically occurs two weeks after your period begins. The sperm and egg meet in one of your fallopian tubes to form a one-celled entity called a zygote. Soon after fertilization, the zygote travels down the fallopian tube to your uterus, where it will burrow into the uterine wall for nourishment.

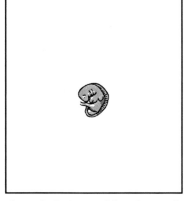

Nerve development is beginning, and your baby has a spinal cord. Primary blood vessels along the central nervous system are now connecting. The eyes and other features begin to form, as well as tiny buds that will become the arms and legs. The heart also forms and begins to beat on the 25th day after conception. Your baby measures about a quarter-inch long and weighs less than one gram, the weight of a 1-ml dropper of water.

Month 2

Your baby's development is very rapid in this month. By the end of month two, all the baby's major organ and body systems have begun to develop. The heartbeat can be detected by ultrasound; however, it will not be possible to hear it at this time. Cells are forming in the neural tube of the brain. Fingers, toes, and sex organs are developing as well. Either labia

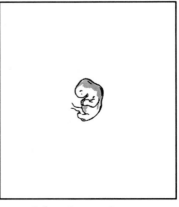

or a penis will begin to form. The jaw and facial muscles are now developing. Tooth buds are also forming at this time. The baby is moving around, but you will not feel anything just yet. Your baby is still less than an inch long and weighs less than two grams.

Month 3

The baby's basic brain structure is now complete, and the nervous system continues to develop. The fingers and toes are more formed and have tiny nails. Hair follicles have started to form on the baby's head, and tooth buds have formed under the baby's gums. The umbilical cord will be fully formed by the end of this month. Your baby's heart now has

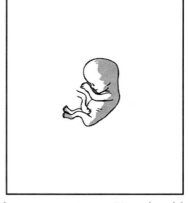

four chambers and beats 120–160 beats per minute. You should be able to hear the baby's heartbeat during this month with a Doppler. The kidneys have developed and are draining urine into the bladder. Vocal cords form, and the baby can make sounds. Any disturbance from drugs, viruses, or toxins may cause birth defects if encountered this month. By the end of month three, all of the baby's major organs are developed. Your baby is about three inches long and weighs about half an ounce.

Month 4

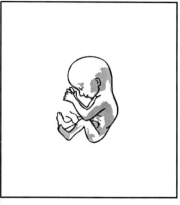

Your baby's face continues to develop. It may have some hair on its head, and teeth begin to form. Eyebrows and eyelashes begin to appear. Buds on the side of the head begin to form into the outer ear. Your baby's digestive system is forming, and the intestines are present. Your baby moves, sleeps, and passes urine. The baby's skin is covered with fine hair called lanugo. By the end of this month, he or she will be between five and six inches long and will weigh about four ounces.

Month 5

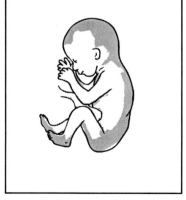

Your baby is growing muscle and becoming stronger. The internal organs are maturing, and your baby now has some fat under its skin. The baby's fingerprints and footprints are now developed. The ears are now developed, and the baby may be able to hear you. Vernix caseosa, a white lanolin-like covering, appears on the baby to protect the skin. Your baby sleeps and eats at regular intervals. The baby can now swallow and might suck its thumb. During this month, you should be able to find out the sex of your baby. By the end of this month, you should be able to feel the baby when it moves inside you. The baby is now about 10 inches long and weighs about 11 ounces.

Month 6

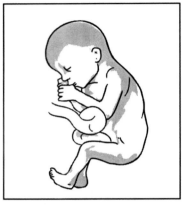

Your baby's brain is developing rapidly, and its bones are becoming solid. Your baby's immune system is developing and will create its own antibodies. You may feel the baby hiccup this month. Your baby is almost fully formed; however, the lungs are still not well developed. The baby is moving amniotic fluid in and out of its lungs. Meconium, your baby's first stool, is developing. By the end of this month, your baby will be 11–14 inches long and weigh 1–1½ pounds.

Month 7

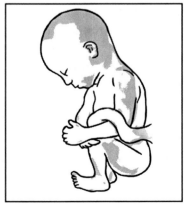

Your baby is continuing to grow and develop. The baby's eyes can now open and close as well as sense changes in light. Your baby can hear much better now; try to talk to it often so that it gets to know your voice. The layer of soft, downy hair called lanugo is starting to disappear from the baby's face. Your baby moves and kicks a lot now and likes to suck its thumb. At this time, the baby may practice breathing. By the end of this month, the baby is about 16 inches long and weighs 2½–3 pounds.

Month 8

You should be feeling strong, regular fetal activity. Your baby continues to put on pounds and store fat all over its body. The lanugo is falling off, and your baby's sucking muscles are ready for action. The baby will have turned head down by this time, in preparation for delivery. At the end of this month, the baby is 16–18 inches long and weighs 4½–5½ pounds.

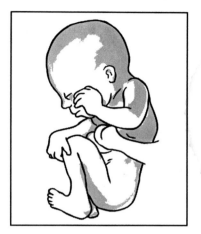

 ## Month 9

Your baby is fully formed, and its lungs are now mature. Your baby is getting fatter and its skin more taut. Even though there isn't much room, the baby will continue to kick until you deliver. If you are having a boy, the testicles should descend. The bones of the baby's head remain soft and flexible to ease its way through the birth canal, and the placenta continues to supply your baby with antibodies that will help fight infection after birth. The baby will continue to gain an ounce a day until you deliver. Your baby is now about 20 inches long and will weigh between six and nine pounds at birth.

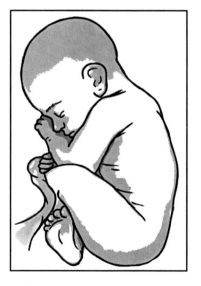

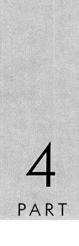

4
PART

STAYING HEALTHY

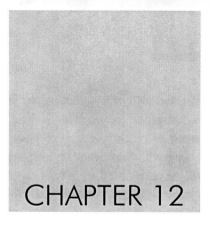

CHAPTER 12

Prenatal Visits

The purpose of prenatal care is to monitor the progress of your pregnancy and to deal with any potential problems that may arise before they become serious for you or your baby. You should call your healthcare provider as soon as you find out you are pregnant. Each provider may have a different time they want to see you for your first visit. You will probably be seen between seven and nine weeks' gestation.

 ## Your First Prenatal Visit

During your first prenatal visit, you will be asked for the details of your complete medical history, including any medications you are presently taking. You will be asked about any prior pregnancies as well as your gynecologic history. You will also be asked to provide your family history of any medical problems or conditions.

You will likely have a complete physical, which includes checking your blood pressure, urine, and weight. A pelvic exam will be performed, and if you haven't had a pap smear recently, one will be done. Prenatal blood work will be performed to assess your blood type and blood count for any evidence of anemia as well as a basic screening to assess your general health. A viral screening will be performed to see if you are immune to rubella, hepatitis, and chickenpox, and, with your consent, you will be tested for HIV. You will also be checked to see if you are a carrier for cystic fibrosis, a hereditary disease. If this is positive, your partner will also need to be checked.

Your delivery date will be determined by the first day of your last period and will be confirmed by your first ultrasound, which is often done at your first prenatal visit. If you have not been taking prenatal vitamins, you will be given a prescription, and these should be taken immediately.

Subsequent Prenatal Visits

Subsequent visits are usually every four weeks until 30 weeks' gestation. You will then be seen every two weeks till the 36th week, and then weekly until delivery (around week 40). If you are seeing a high-risk specialist during your pregnancy, you may be seen more frequently.

Most of these visits involve checking your weight, blood pressure, and urine. Your belly will be measured to check the baby's growth. The doctor will listen to the baby's heartbeat, which can usually be heard after 10 weeks' gestation. You will also be asked about any problems or concerns you are having.

Once you start seeing your provider on a regular basis, you should keep a running list of questions and concerns to bring to each scheduled visit so that you don't forget them once you get there. On the other hand, if something doesn't feel right to you in your body, and you are concerned about it, pick up the phone and call your doctor's office. It is always better to be safe than sorry. Doctors expect their pregnant patients to have many questions, and they will do their very best to answer all of them.

It is important to remember that your physician/caregiver is not only caring for you, but also for your unborn baby. The medical decisions being made by your doctor are to ensure the best possible outcome for both mother and child. If you have any questions related to how your care is being handled, let your healthcare provider know that you need a little extra time to go over your concerns and desires.

Good communication between you and your practitioner is key to a successful pregnancy!

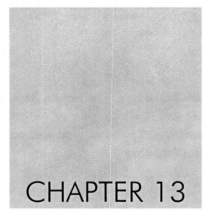

CHAPTER 13

Eating Healthy During Your Pregnancy

The benefits of eating a healthy diet are numerous when you are pregnant. Studies show that maintaining a healthy diet from the beginning of your pregnancy will reduce complications that may occur in the second and third trimesters.

The term "eating for two" is often misunderstood by pregnant women. Eating for two does not mean eating twice as much. The recommended caloric intake for a woman in her childbearing years who is not pregnant is 2,000 calories a day. A pregnant woman needs only an extra 300 calories a day in her second and third trimesters. Extra calories are not really needed in the first trimester of pregnancy. An extra 300 calories a day is not that much food. Eating a piece of fruit and a cup of yogurt could easily equal 300 calories. Of course, if you are involved in an exercise program, you could get away with some extra calories per day without it making much difference.

It is normal to have an increased appetite when you are pregnant. The best way to handle this increased hunger is with smaller, more frequent meals. Eating in this manner will also ensure that your blood sugar doesn't get too low. Having low blood sugar can cause dizziness, headaches, and nausea.

 ## Dietary Recommendations for Pregnant Women

Protein: You need to eat three servings of protein per day. Protein is found in animal and dairy products. Other sources of protein include whole grains, seeds, nuts, dried beans (cooked), and tofu.

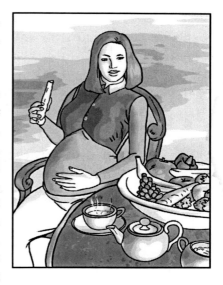

Carbohydrates: There are two kinds of carbohydrates: simple and complex. Simple carbs, such as cookies and candy, are high in sugar and should be very limited in your diet. They offer little value to you and your health. The main exception is fruit (see below), which contains fructose and is much better for you. Complex carbs are found in starchy foods like breads, pasta, rice, potatoes, and legumes. Eat between four and six servings per day of these.

Dairy: Have at least four servings per day. Milk, cheese, and yogurt are all good sources of calcium. Skim milk or 1 percent are preferable, as these products have the same amount of calcium without the higher calories associated with whole milk's fat content.

Fats: Your fat intake should not exceed 30 percent of your daily consumption of food. Most fats should come from unsaturated sources, such as fish, nuts, and oils like olive, canola, and sunflower. Omega-3 fatty acids are also beneficial fats to be included in your diet. These fats can be found in oily fishes, such as salmon and sardines. Nuts, such as walnuts, and flaxseed contain this type of fat as well.

Fruits: You should have between two and four servings a day. Your fruits can also be consumed in juice form. Dried fruits are also a good low-calorie snack.

Vegetables: You should have at least four servings per day. Your vegetables can be eaten raw or cooked. Salads are always a great low-calorie meal.

Water: You should be drinking at least eight glasses of water a day.

 ## Vitamin and Mineral Recommendations for Pregnant Women

Many women do not get enough of certain vitamins and minerals from food, so taking a good prenatal vitamin that includes folic acid and iron is recommended. Folic acid reduces the risk of spina bifida (open spine in the baby), and iron protects you from developing anemia during your pregnancy.

An alternative would be to take any over-the-counter, balanced multivitamin that includes 400–600 micrograms of folic acid and a 27-mg iron supplement. Folic acid and small amounts of iron can also be found in foods like spinach, broccoli, lentils, asparagus, orange juice, romaine lettuce, and enriched breads and pastas.

 ## Foods and Drinks That Should Be Avoided in Pregnancy

Because certain foods can contain harmful bacteria or are known to be unsafe during pregnancy, it is best to take precautions to make sure they are safe to eat or to avoid them altogether.

- Avoid fish that is high in mercury, such as shark, swordfish, mackerel, and tilefish. Albacore tuna *can* be eaten, but should be limited to once a week.
- Avoid unpasteurized soft cheeses, such as brie, feta, and blue cheese.
- Avoid eggs that are not thoroughly cooked or any foods that contain raw eggs.

o Avoid unpasteurized milk or any foods made from it.

o Avoid raw shellfish.

o Caffeine should be kept to a minimum.

o Avoid raw sprouts.

o Avoid raw or undercooked meat and chicken.

o Deli meats and hot dogs should be avoided unless they are reheated.

o Saccharin is an artificial sweetener that should not be consumed during pregnancy because it has been shown to cross the placenta. Other artificial sweeteners can be used in moderation.

o Avoid unwashed vegetables.

o Alcoholic beverages should be avoided, especially in the first trimester.

Weight Gain during Pregnancy

As you probably know, gaining weight during pregnancy is normal, but if you are already overweight, your total gain may be as little as 10–15 pounds for a healthy pregnancy. Recent studies have shown that obese women do not need to gain any weight during pregnancy and can actually lose a few pounds without any harm to the baby. If you are of normal weight, your recommended weight gain should be 25–35 pounds. If you are underweight, it is recommended you gain 28–40 pounds. If you are carrying twins and are at a healthy weight, you should gain 35–45 pounds.

On average, a pregnant woman can expect to gain about three pounds in the first trimester, 10–12 pounds in the second trimester, and 10–15 pounds in the third trimester. Please see table 13.1 to see how this weight gain breaks down between you and your baby.

Table 13.1: Breakdown of Pregnancy Weight Gain

Baby	7½ lbs
Placenta	1½ lbs
Amniotic Fluid	2 lbs
Mother's Fat Stores	5–6 lbs
Increased Blood Volume	3 lbs
Water Increase	5 lbs
Breasts	1 lb
Uterus	2 lbs

 Steps you can take to ensure a normal healthy weight gain during your pregnancy:

○ Eat three meals a day with two to three snacks in between.

○ Watch your portion sizes.

○ Stick to broiled and grilled foods, and stay away from deep-fried foods.

○ Stay away from fast food.

○ Stay away from junk food with empty calories.

○ Carry healthy snacks with you in case you get hungry.

○ Exercise a few days a week.

What is a BMI?

Body mass index (BMI) is a measurement that healthcare providers use to evaluate your weight and discuss healthcare issues related to it. A recommended BMI is in the 19–25 range.

If you weigh more than 200 pounds or your BMI is 30 or over, you should see a doctor (family physician or ob/gyn) before you get pregnant. It is important to discuss your potential risks and how you can plan for a healthy pregnancy. Low BMIs (under 19) can also be associated with risks, including a small baby and a preterm birth.

Please see table 13.2 to find your BMI on the chart.

Table 13.2: Body Mass Index by Height and Weight

	Healthy		Overweight		Obese		
BMI➔	19	24	25	29	30	35	40
Height	Weight						
4' 10"	91	115	119	138	143	167	191
4' 11"	94	119	124	143	148	173	198
5' 0"	97	123	128	148	153	179	204
5' 1"	100	127	132	153	158	185	211
5' 1"	104	131	136	158	164	191	218
5' 3"	107	135	141	163	169	197	225
5' 4"	110	140	145	169	174	204	232
5' 5"	114	144	150	174	180	210	240
5' 6"	118	148	1558	179	186	216	247
5' 7"	121	153	159	185	191	223	255
5' 8"	125	158	164	190	197	230	262
5' 9"	128	162	169	196	203	236	270
5' 10"	132	167	174	202	209	243	278
5' 11"	136	172	179	208	215	250	286
6' 0"	140	177	184	213	221	258	294

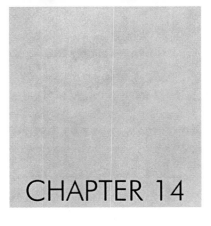

CHAPTER 14

Exercise and Pregnancy

Exercising during pregnancy can be very beneficial. It can help prepare you for labor and delivery, and it will help you get back to pre-pregnancy shape sooner. Many forms of exercise are considered safe during pregnancy. Whether you have been exercising regularly or are thinking about starting an exercise routine, you should talk to your healthcare provider to make sure you do not have any obstetric or health conditions that would restrict activity. Your provider might advise against exercising if you have risk factors for preterm labor or develop a problem during the pregnancy, such as vaginal bleeding.

 ## Safe exercises during pregnancy include:

- ○ **Walking:** a full body workout that is great exercise for anyone.

- ○ **Swimming:** it's easy on your joints and keeps you from overheating.

- ○ **Aerobics**: if you limit it to low impact, it's great for cardiovascular health.

- ○ **Treadmill:** set on a gentle incline and decreased speed, it offers the same great benefits as walking.

o **Strength Training:** with use of low weights, it might help ease aches and pains.

o **Prenatal Pilates:** it's great for building core strength to help push that baby out.

o **Yoga:** it helps with relaxation and breathing for a natural childbirth experience.

 ## Activities that should be avoided during pregnancy include:

o Any contact sport

o Snow skiing

o Scuba diving

o Horseback riding

o Any activity that involves jumping

After the first trimester, exercises should be avoided that require you to lie flat on your back. The expanding uterus causes pressure on the vena cava, the large vein that carries blood back to the heart, reducing blood flow to both the mother and the baby.

If your gym has a hot tub or steam room, it is best to avoid them during pregnancy. Their use can raise your body temperature to a dangerous level. In addition, a high body temperature can cause a woman's blood pressure to fall, which could result in less oxygen to the baby.

 ## Keep in mind the following tips when exercising while pregnant:

o All exercising should be done in moderation.

o Thirty minutes of exercise a day is plenty to keep in shape.

o Begin any workout with a warm-up period of 5–10

minutes, and follow it with by a cool-down period of 5–10 minutes.

o   Avoid performing any exercise in very hot and humid weather, as you are more at risk for overheating.

o   Drink plenty of fluids to keep from getting dehydrated and overheated.

o   Know your limitations.

 You should discontinue exercising if you experience any of the following symptoms:

o   Dizziness

o   Shortness of breath or chest pain

o   Fluid leaking from vagina

o   Vaginal bleeding

o   Uterine contractions

If these symptoms do not subside after a short while, contact your healthcare provider promptly.

CHAPTER 15

Immunizations and Vaccines

Vaccines are medicines that can be given to help protect you from various diseases. They are made from killed or weakened viruses. Vaccines will cause your body's immune system to make antibodies. Once these antibodies are present, they protect you if you are exposed to that disease in the future. If you are at an increased risk for infection, your doctor may suggest that you get vaccinated for certain diseases and avoid vaccinations for others.

 The following vaccines should be given to all expectant moms at a higher risk of exposure:

○ Hepatitis B
○ Influenza
○ Diphtheria
○ Tetanus
○ Rabies
○ Pneumococcal
○ Meningococcal

The following vaccines contain a live virus and should be avoided during pregnancy even if you are at a higher risk of exposure:

- Measles
- Mumps
- Rubella
- Varicella (chickenpox)
- Lyme disease
- Nasal spray flu vaccine
- BCG (tuberculosis)
- Human papillomavirus

 ## Some Additional Comments

Varicella (chickenpox)

The effects of the varicella vaccine on a developing fetus remain unknown. It is recommended that pregnancy should be avoided for three months after receiving the vaccine. If a pregnant woman gets this virus in the second or third trimester, up to 2 percent of fetuses can be affected, with mild to severe outcomes. Contact your doctor if you think you may have been exposed.

Tetanus/Diphtheria

If Mom is at risk and has not recently been immunized, she should get immunized, as there is no risk to the fetus from the immunization. There is great risk to both mother and baby if she is exposed during the pregnancy, however.

Lyme Disease

Lyme disease is transmitted through a deer tick bite. The first sign of an infection is a circular rash that resembles a bull's-eye. Some people may also experience flu-like symptoms. If you find a tick on your body, you should remove it with a pair of tweezers.

Your doctor should be contacted if you find a tick on your body or think you have been bitten by one, as testing may be available to determine if you have been infected. Studies of women infected during pregnancy have found that, if treated with the appropriate antibiotic, there is no negative effect to the fetus.

CHAPTER 16

Drugs and Toxic Exposures to the Fetus

 ## Medication

It is rare that a pregnant woman will go through her pregnancy without needing some type of over-the-counter medication, and sometimes, she will even need a prescription medication. Fortunately, many over-the-counter and prescription drugs are safe to take in pregnancy.

The FDA has categorized drugs into five categories that apply to pregnancy:

- **Category A** drugs have shown no risk to the fetus.
- **Category B** drugs are generally considered safe to take in pregnancy.
- **Category C** drugs should be given only if the potential benefit justifies the potential risk to the fetus.
- **Category D** drugs show evidence of human fetal risk. The benefits from use in pregnant women may be acceptable despite the risk.
- **Category X** drugs are never to be taken by women who are or may become pregnant.

The most dangerous time to expose the fetus to drugs or toxic agents is between five and 12 weeks of pregnancy. After the first trimester, the baby's major organ systems are developed, and it is considered a much safer time to take medication.

It should be noted that the use of regular-strength aspirin and non-steroidal, anti-inflammatory drugs (NSAIDs) like ibuprofen (Aleve and Motrin, for example) should generally be avoided during pregnancy. The use of aspirin in the first trimester can increase the risk of miscarriage, and use in the third trimester is not recommended due to the fact that aspirin can change your blood's ability to clot. This could be dangerous during and following delivery. Women taking low-dose (81-mg) aspirin throughout pregnancy for specific antibody disorders are not at any increased risk for these types of problems.

Non-steroidal, anti-inflammatory drugs should be avoided especially during the third trimester of pregnancy. Use of these drugs can cause a premature closure of the ductus arteriosus (a vessel in the fetal heart), which can lead to high blood pressure in the fetal lungs. This can be dangerous to the baby's health after birth.

Check with your doctor about any medications you may need to take during the pregnancy.

 ## Smoking during Pregnancy

In the United States, more than 18 percent of women smoke. Recent studies have shown that 7 percent of pregnant women are smokers. Cigarette smoke contains more than 2,500 harmful chemicals. Both nicotine and carbon monoxide can cause many adverse pregnancy outcomes.

Risks related to smoking while pregnant include:
- ○ Two times greater risk of low-birth-weight babies
- ○ Increased risk of mental retardation
- ○ Increased risk of learning disabilities

o   Increased risk of respiratory diseases

o   Increased risk of preterm birth

o   Increased risk of cleft lip/palate

o   Increased risk of ectopic pregnancy

o   Increased risk of placenta previa

o   Increased risk of placental abruption

o   Increased risk of infertility

The more a woman smokes, the more likely she is to have a low-birth-weight baby. However, if a woman stops smoking in her second trimester of pregnancy, she is no more likely to have a low-birth-weight baby than a woman who never smoked.

Studies have also shown that a woman who smokes one month prior to getting pregnant up to the end of her first trimester has a greater risk of having a baby with birth defects, especially congenital heart defects. There can be other long-term health risks for your baby as well: more colds, lung problems, learning disabilities, and physical growth problems.

Babies whose mothers smoke during pregnancy undergo withdrawal-like symptoms much like babies of mothers who use drugs as dangerous as heroin and cocaine. *A baby is also three times more likely to die from sudden infant death syndrome (SIDS) than babies whose mothers do not smoke.*

So, if you smoke and you are pregnant now or planning to become pregnant, it is especially important to kick the habit now. You can ask your doctor for ways to help you quit, including information on which smoking cessation aids are safe for you and your baby and how you can get in touch with quitting programs in the area. Many community organizations and some hospitals sponsor such programs.

According to the American Lung Association, new studies have shown that if a pregnant woman is around secondhand smoke, the risks are still significant.

X-ray Exposure

Most x-rays that adults are exposed to carry a very low risk of danger to the fetus. The fetus needs three to five rads of x-ray exposure to have an increased risk of leukemia (equivalent to 40–50 chest x-rays). A chest x-ray causes an exposure of one-tenth of a rad to the mother, with an even lower amount of x-ray exposure to the fetus, and is very safe. Dental x-rays, with a lead apron shield covering the front of your body, cause no detectable x-ray exposure to the fetus and are safe if needed for evaluation of the mother by a dentist.

 ## Caffeine

Caffeine is a stimulant that is present in many drinks. Many of us love a cup of coffee or soda, which may contain caffeine. The diuretic effect of caffeine increases the risk of washing out calcium and other nutrients needed during your pregnancy. You also urinate more frequently after consuming caffeine, which can result in dehydration. Caffeine circulates for many hours in the fetal compartment after it has washed through your body. This can be associated with premature atrial contractions (PACs) in the fetal heart that can put stress on the fetus. Preferably, you should keep your caffeine intake to a minimum, with an occasional cup of coffee, but not daily.

 ## Hair Products

There are no studies showing a relationship between the use of hair colorings, straighteners, or other hair products and birth defects in the fetus. However, to be on the safe side, you should avoid use of these products until all organ systems of the fetus are completely formed at 12 weeks' gestation. These products are fine to use in the second and third trimesters.

Household Cleaners

Normal household cleaners have not been shown to cause harm to a developing fetus. All pregnant women should read labels carefully and avoid using any cleaners that say they contain toxic chemicals. You should also be aware of labels that warn you to use a product only in a well-ventilated area. This most likely means that the product emits very strong fumes. If you are concerned about the use of commercial cleaners, you can use one of the many new cleaning products on the market today that are environmentally friendly. When using any cleaner, you should always wear rubber gloves to protect your skin.

 ## Alcohol

Exposure to alcohol has been associated with fetal heart abnormalities, facial malformations, low birth weight, and learning disabilities (fetal alcohol syndrome). If you have had a drink or two during your pregnancy, the odds are that your baby will be fine, but it is still best to avoid alcoholic beverages while pregnant.

 ## Illicit Drugs

Exposure to any illicit drug is dangerous to your unborn baby. If you are using drugs throughout your pregnancy, the baby will most likely suffer through withdrawal after being born. Exposure to cocaine can be associated with stillbirth, fetal heart disease, placental abruption, and small babies.

CHAPTER 17

Working during Your Pregnancy

With more women working outside of home, the number of pregnant women in the workplace has increased dramatically. Pregnancy in the workplace is much more accepted these days, especially with the number of women in high-position jobs. Even so, many women still worry about breaking the news to their employers.

If you work full-time and are not sure that you want to return to your full-time position, you should discuss with your employer what options are available to you. Your employer may be willing to let you work part-time hours or, if possible, let you work from home. Even if your employer agrees only to let you make an alternative arrangement for a certain period of time, this could be a situation that will work for you.

If you still plan to work full-time after the baby is born, be sure to let your employer know this. It is important that employers know your job is still a priority for you even though you will be gone for a short while.

When is work a potential hazard to your pregnancy?

The answer is usually never. However, some work requires strenuous lifting or long periods of standing or walking that can increase the risk of preterm labor and a smaller than normal baby. If you are exposed to hazardous chemicals or toxic substances at work, this can be harmful to your baby and should be discussed with your doctor. Working in the medical field can potentially expose you to certain infections. Wearing gloves and washing your hands often is always recommended.

If you have a complicated pregnancy that may require you to rest more than usual, have your obstetrician or healthcare provider write a note to your employer stating what your limitations are in the workplace.

Steps you can take to stay safe and healthy while working:

- ○ Make sure not to skip any meals.
- ○ Drink plenty of fluids.
- ○ Make sure to empty your bladder regularly.
- ○ If you have a desk job, make sure to get up and walk around every few hours.
- ○ Avoid lifting heavy objects if possible.
- ○ Get at least seven hours of sleep each night.
- ○ Be careful when using steps, especially in the third trimester when you can no longer see the ground.

The following complications may affect your ability to work:

- ○ Hypertension
- ○ Diabetes
- ○ Severe nausea and vomiting
- ○ Multiple gestation
- ○ Growth-restricted gestation
- ○ Morbid obesity
- ○ Advanced maternal age (over 35 years old)
- ○ Bleeding (vaginally) during your pregnancy

- o Premature labor
- o Low amniotic fluid (oligohydramnios)
- o Mild preeclampsia
- o Cervical incompetence

Pregnancy Rights in the Workplace

Prior to informing your employer that you are expecting, take time to get familiar with what a pregnant woman's rights are in the workplace. The information regarding these laws can be obtained through your human resource department at work. You can also check the Internet for specific laws that may apply to your state.

The Pregnancy Discrimination Act of 1978 prohibits an employer from discriminating against you because you are pregnant or for any medical condition related to your pregnancy. This law states that employers must treat you as they would any other employee with a medical disability.

In addition, The Family Medical Leave Act (FMLA) is a federal law that applies to any employee who works on a workforce of 50 or more employees. If you have worked for such a company for more than one year, you are permitted to take up to 12 weeks of unpaid leave for various family and medical reasons, including childbirth. This law guarantees that upon return to work, your same position or one of equal seniority will be available with the same salary as when you left.

CHAPTER 18

Bed Rest during Pregnancy

Being ordered to bed rest can seem like a pretty good deal at first, especially if you work outside the home. Soon enough, though, reality hits, and you realize that maybe this is not going to be such a picnic after all.

Over 20 percent of all pregnant women delivering in the United States are placed on bed rest for an interval of time. There are many reasons why your doctor may place you on bed rest.

 The most common reasons to be placed on some type of bed rest include:

- o Bleeding in first, second, or third trimesters
- o Preterm contractions
- o A shortened cervix
- o Multiple gestations
- o A small baby
- o High blood pressure

 Types of bed rest that you may be placed on include:

Moderate Bed Rest

Moderate bed rest is a rest period of 1½–2 hours with a half hour of low-level activity before the next rest period. There should be at least three of these rest periods between 8:00 AM and 6:00 PM daily. During this time, you should not lift heavy things (greater than 10 pounds). Driving to a nearby location or running a quick errand is usually permitted. With modified bed rest, most women can take 10-minute walks a couple of times a day.

Strict Bed Rest
Strict bed rest means that you need to be in a horizontal position all day except for trips to use the bathroom. A brief shower is usually fine but taking warm baths is usually not suggested. You may be allowed up for a few minutes to prepare a simple meal, although it would be a good idea to keep snacks and a drink close by so that you do not need to get up too often. You may or may not be allowed to have sexual intercourse during this time. This will depend on the reason you were put on bed rest in the first place. Be sure to check with your provider as to what exactly your limitations are.

Strict bed rest can cause joint pain and backaches because of limited movement. Stretching exercises are strongly suggested.

Managing Your Bed Rest
Even though your activities have been restricted, you can still get many things accomplished during this time. Keeping busy will definitely make the time pass faster.

- If you worked prior to being placed on bed rest, perhaps you can still get some work done with the use of a laptop computer.
- You can still buy many of the things you need for the baby, either through a catalog or online.
- Now may be a good time to read that book you never found the time to read before.
- Take some time to catch up with some friends, either by e-mail or phone.

Support from family and friends can make this time much easier for you—especially if you have other children to take care of. If you can get someone to help out with meal preparation and daily errands, it will be a great relief to you and the rest of your family.

If you have been put on bed rest for a long time, *take it one day at a time only*. Dwelling on how much time you still have left in the pregnancy will only drive you crazy. Think positively that you are doing this for the best possible outcome for your baby. It will be well worth it in the end.

CHAPTER 19

Air Travel and Vacations during Pregnancy

Most women can safely travel during pregnancy. With a little extra planning and precaution, you should not encounter any problems. Just make sure your caregiver is aware of your travel plans beforehand.

 Tips for Safe Vacationing When You Are Pregnant

○ The most common obstetrical emergencies happen in the first and third trimesters. The second trimester is the best time to travel.

○ Enjoy yourself, but be careful when doing new types of physical activities. Pregnancy changes a woman's balance, and her coordination is not as good. Walking and low-risk physical activities are usually fine to participate in and enjoy.

○ Always keep yourself well hydrated during the day because increased activity can cause dehydration. Dehydration can cause your uterus to contract and may mean a trip to a hospital far from home.

○ Avoid tap water and ice cubes in foreign countries. You should drink only bottled water.

- Do not go into the ocean, as this can increase your risk for both vaginal and womb infection, which could result in a premature delivery.
- Always locate a hospital that you can go to when on vacation.
- If possible, you should not travel alone.

 ## Tips for Air Travel during Pregnancy

- Air travel is safe for most women up to 34 weeks of pregnancy.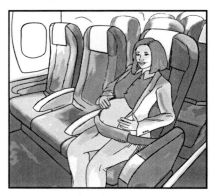
- Each airline has specific rules regarding air travel during pregnancy, so check with the carrier beforehand. Some airlines require a letter from your doctor stating how many weeks pregnant you are at the time of your trip.
- Second- or third-trimester vaginal bleeding, premature labor, pregnancy-induced high blood pressure, type 1 or type 2 diabetes, sickle cell anemia (or trait), and multiple gestation are some reasons that air travel may not be permitted.
- If you get nauseous when flying, anti-nausea medications are suggested. They are safe to take during pregnancy.
- Drink plenty of fluids before you leave, and drink more fluids during the flight. Do not drink lots of carbonated beverages as this can increase the chance of nausea.
- Wear thigh-high support stockings. This will reduce the risk of fluid accumulation in your legs and feet and reduce the risk of blood clots forming in the legs.
- Get up and walk around the cabin once every hour.
- Always use your seat belt *below your belly* when seated.

? I have to travel three hours by air and am almost 37 weeks along. Is there a problem if I tell the airline attendant at the gate that I am a couple of weeks earlier?

Should something happen and you rupture your water bag or go into labor, the jet might have to divert its trip, landing somewhere else to take you to the hospital. If this should occur and the air carrier finds out that you lied about your gestational age, you would be charged the cost of getting you to your emergency care. That could run you between $35,000 and $70,000. I know two couples who had to pay for such an ordeal of diverting the airliner, so I suggest you only fly by the rules!

? What is the best advice you can give me whether my trip is by car, train, boat, or air?

- Relax and enjoy yourself.
- Drink lots of bottled water.
- Do not do any physical activities that could be dangerous.
- Remember to bring along all the medications you are taking.
- Bring a copy of your medical records in case you require any care.
- Locate a medical center that cares for pregnant women near where you are staying.
- Check with your health insurance company to make sure you are covered if you should need care at your destination.
- Use appropriate medication for nausea if necessary.
- Always buckle your seat belt below your belly.
- Walk around for a few minutes every couple of hours when traveling (every hour if by air).
- Wear flat, comfortable shoes.
- Get plenty of rest.

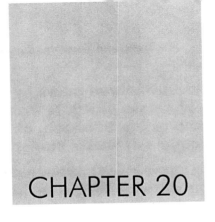

CHAPTER 20

Sex during Pregnancy

Women and men never know how pregnancy will influence their sexual relationship until it happens. Many women who have nausea and feel sick in the first trimester have little interest in having sex or being physically intimate. In addition, some men fear that having sex will cause an early miscarriage. While it is true that a woman's desire for having sex usually decreases in the first trimester, first trimester losses are not caused by sexual intercourse.

With changes in hormone levels that occur throughout pregnancy, the second trimester is the time the average woman says she enjoys sex the most. The nausea is gone, she feels emotionally and physically the best, and her body is not as swollen and awkward in movement as it is in the third trimester. Many women find that during pregnancy they can have orgasms faster and more often during lovemaking. This is due to an increase in blood flow to the clitoris and vagina.

A woman's changing body shape can be a turn-on or turn-off for either partner. A couple may need to explore different positions during sex to enjoy physical intimacy. Being open, honest, and having a good sense of humor during this time will make the experience more relaxed and satisfying for each partner. For women who have restrictions placed upon them related to intercourse, oral sex and mutual masturbation can be just as satisfying for both partners. Oral sex is permissible during pregnancy, but your partner should be aware that blowing into the vagina is dangerous. Sometimes, just talking and massaging one another can also be an enjoyable experience.

Men are often fearful that the penis in the vagina can hurt the baby or cause preterm labor. Women with an uncomplicated pregnancy do not need to worry about this happening. Movements of the baby during and after sex are normal. Some couples have asked if the baby can know and remember that Mom and Dad had sex. The answer is, of course, no. You should just enjoy each other and forget about the little one in there along for the ride!

Many women have a little bit of bleeding following intercourse, but this is normal and usually comes from the cervix. You do not need to call your doctor unless it becomes heavier and is causing uncomfortable contractions as well.

If you have pregnancy complications, talk with your doctor about sex and what you can and cannot do. The main problems limiting sex include cervical incompetence, preterm labor, and placental abruption or placenta previa.

If you do not have any complications during your pregnancy, just enjoy yourself, remembering that with increased blood flow, your orgasms will be stronger and more frequent. So, have some fun!

5
PART

Fetal Evaluation during Pregnancy

CHAPTER 21

Causes of Birth Defects

About 98 percent of newborns each year are born with no serious birth defects. That means two out of 100 newborns—or 100,000 babies per year—will be born in the United States with a mild to serious birth defect or genetic abnormality.

A birth defect is an abnormality that is present from the moment of birth. These abnormalities can be inherited genetically from either the mother or the father. They can also be caused by a birth injury or acquired during the course of the pregnancy.

Genetics is the passing of human characteristics from generation to generation. We have 3 billion DNA base pairs determining who we are. Everyone has about 100,000 genes made up of many DNA base pairs that give us our unique characteristics. We normally have 22 pairs of chromosomes in each cell, which contain thousands of genes. In addition, we have a pair of sex chromosomes—either XX female or XY male.

 ## Autosomal Dominant Disorders

In an autosomal *dominant* disorder, only one mutated copy of the gene is necessary for a person to be affected. That means that only one of the parents may be mildly or severely affected. Any child that you have has a 50 percent chance of receiving that dominant gene and being affected. Examples of these disorders include Huntington's disease, neurofibromatosis, and Marfan syndrome.

 ## Autosomal Recessive Disorders

In autosomal *recessive* disorders, two copies of the gene must be mutated for a person to be affected. Both parents must have a copy of such an abnormal gene. Two unaffected parents who carry the gene have a one in four, or 25 percent, chance of passing the gene to their child. If the child gets the affected gene from each parent, the child will have the disease. All unborn children can be tested by chorionic villus sampling (CVS) or amniocentesis to see if they have the disease. The most commonly tested recessive diseases include cystic fibrosis, sickle cell anemia, and Tay-Sachs.

Diseases on the X and Y chromosomes follow the same inheritance patterns.

 ## Chromosome-Related Birth Defects

All men and women have 46 chromosomes. A chromosomal abnormality occurs when the egg and sperm do not divide equally. The most well-known risk factor for this to occur is the age of the egg or the age of the mother. Studies have recently shown that if the father is over the age of 50 there is also a risk factor.

 ## The following are risk factors for genetic disorders:

- Being over the age of 35 when your baby is due
- A family history of neural tube defects
- A family history of Down syndrome or other chromosome disorders
- A history of sickle cell anemia
- Family history of congenital heart disease

- o Family history of unknown origin for mental retardation
- o Tay-Sachs history or being of Jewish descent
- o Family treatment for fragile X syndrome
- o Any rare metabolic disorders or type 1 juvenile diabetes
- o History of a stillbirth
- o More than two miscarriages in a row
- o Family history of muscular dystrophy
- o Family history of hemophilia

If you have a checkmark on any of the factors listed above, let your doctor know that you want to have genetic counseling. It is very important that you get this counseling *before* you become pregnant. If you do not have any of these risk factors but are still concerned about the possibility of having a child with a genetic disorder, you should consult with a genetic counselor.

Congenital heart disease, spina bifida, cleft lip/palate, and clubfoot are caused by a combination of factors called *multifactorial inheritance.* The actual causes are unknown, but we think they have a higher risk of occurring in families that carry an inherited risk higher than the general population for these birth defects.

Congenital heart disease is the most common birth defect, occurring in one in 130 births, and 30–40 percent of babies with these heart defects have a chromosomal problem. It is important for *all* pregnant women to have a level 2 or anatomical ultrasound by a physician specially trained in detecting abnormalities in babies by that method.

If you have had a prior pregnancy that was diagnosed with a chromosomal abnormality, the chance of having another is 1 percent. If your family has a very rare chromosome disorder where two chromosomes are connected to each other, 20–30 percent of all children can have a serious chromosome defect.

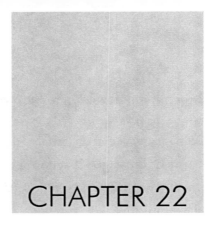

CHAPTER 22

Prenatal Diagnosis

There is no doubt that the most common question asked by couples is, "Does my baby look normal?" Along with the feelings of anticipation, excitement, and joy, come concerns about the baby's health.

Technology has advanced in the last 25 years to help a woman get a better idea of what her chances are of having a baby with a chromosomal abnormality or birth defect, but first it is important to understand what exactly these tests do and what they mean.

There are two types of prenatal tests: screening tests and diagnostic tests.

 ## Screening Tests

Screening tests do not diagnose problems, they simply evaluate risk. These tests give you a result that says your risk is either high or low for having a baby with a chromosomal abnormality or neural tube defect. Screening test results range from one in 10 (very high) to one in 10,000 (very low). If your result shows a higher risk than one in 270, such as one in 250, your risk would be greater than a woman who is age 35 or older. If your risk is less than one in 270, such as one in 290, this would mean that you are not in a high-risk category for having a baby with a chromosomal abnormality. The main purpose of a screening test in pregnancy is to give an expectant mother a heads-up as to whether the risk is increased for having a baby with a chromosomal abnormality.

The screening tests you will be offered include the following:

Nuchal Translucency

A nuchal translucency (NT) test is done between 11 and 13 weeks' gestation. This test is performed by ultrasound and measures the thickness of the back of the baby's neck. If the nuchal translucency—the space at the back of the developing baby's neck—is thicker than average, there is a higher risk for chromosomal abnormalities and congenital heart disease. Depending on the timing of the scan, a normal NT measurement is between 2 mm and 3 mm or less.

If the findings are abnormal, you should be counseled at that time on your options for diagnostic testing. The fetus should also have a fetal echocardiogram and cardiac evaluation between 18 and 22 weeks' gestation with a pediatric cardiologist.

PAPP-A

This is a blood test done on the expectant mom at the same time the NT screening test is done. The PAPP-A, combined with the nuchal translucency measurement, will calculate your risk of having a baby with a chromosomal abnormality. If the NT measurement is calculated incorrectly by the individual performing the study, the PAPP-A result may be inaccurate.

Triple Screen/Quad Screen

The triple screen is a blood test done in the mid-second trimester that measures alpha-fetoprotein (MSAFP), human chorionic gonadotropin (hCG), and estriol. This test is used for determining a risk for chromosomal abnormalities, such as Down syndrome and spinal abnormalities like spina bifida.

The quad screen is another blood panel performed in the

mid-second trimester. This test will identify up to 85 percent of women who have a higher risk for carrying a baby with a chromosomal abnormality. This means that 15 percent of women carrying a baby with a chromosomal abnormality will not be identified.

Integrated Screening

This test combines the NT ultrasound measurement with the PAPP-A blood test and the second-trimester blood test. A risk is not given to the patient concerning chromosomal abnormalities until the quad screen is done in the second trimester.

I believe that the largest percentage of women who are at risk for chromosomal abnormalities will be found with the integrated test. However, if the first trimester NT measurement is abnormal, the mother should be offered a CVS procedure rather than waiting until the second quad screen is finished at 17–19 weeks. If a CVS is not offered at this time, you should request it.

Can a screening test ever produce a false-positive result?

This is not possible because a screening test can never diagnose a chromosomal abnormality. Often, a woman who is told that her testing is "positive" or "abnormal" will take this to mean that the baby will most likely have an abnormality. This is not true. It only means that you have been put into a higher-risk category. Of course, this will certainly cause any woman a lot of worry, most often unnecessary.

Ultrasound-Limited (Level 1)

Ultrasound is a harmless procedure that uses sound waves to create a picture of your baby on a screen. A limited ultrasound can be performed in the first, second, or third trimester and will most likely be done at your obstetrician's office. An ultrasound performed in the early first trimester is usually done for dating a pregnancy or checking if the pregnancy is viable. Often, because the baby is very small at this stage, a transvaginal ultrasound will be done. This is because an abdominal ultrasound cannot offer good visualization very early in pregnancy. Limited ultrasounds performed throughout pregnancy are used to check the basic anatomy of the baby, growth, amniotic fluid, the mother's cervix, and the position of the baby. In addition, at 15–22 weeks' gestation, "soft markers" are looked for that might indicate a higher risk of chromosomal abnormalities.

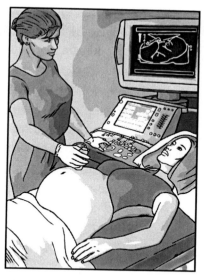

"Soft markers" that can increase your risk for chromosome abnormalities include:

- ○ **Intracardiac echogenic focus (ICEF)** is a small calcium fleck in the fetal heart and can increase the risk for Down syndrome by two to three times more than the patient's age-related risks. If the fetus has normal chromosomes from an amniocentesis, there are no short- or long-term risks for the fetus from this small fleck of calcium.

- ○ **Choroid plexus cyst (CPC)** is a small, fluid-filled cyst in an area of the fetal brain called the choroid plexus. This can increase the risk of chromosomal abnormalities, specifically Trisomy 18. If the fetus has normal chromosomes, these cysts are usually benign and pose no risk to the fetus. Most of the time, these cysts disappear by 28 weeks' gestation. However, if the fetus has choroid plexus cysts on each side of the brain that are larger than 10 mm, there is a greater likelihood of a neurological problem. Further testing would be necessary, and a consultation with a pediatric neurologist would be recommended.

- o **Hydronephrosis** is an accumulation of fluid in the fetal kidneys and is a common finding in males. This can increase the risk of chromosomal abnormalities.

- o **Echogenic bowel** is a brightness of the bowel seen by ultrasound. The brightness comes from a slowing of fecal material moving through the bowel, or swallowing of blood or mucus by the baby. The risk of a chromosomal abnormality being present can depend on the brightness of the echogenic bowel as seen on ultrasound. This finding can increase your risk for Down syndrome and other chromosomal abnormalities. This finding can also be associated with cystic fibrosis. If all diagnostic tests are normal, then this finding is usually insignificant.

- o **Short femur bones**—more than 10 days shorter than the mean gestational age—increases the risk for Down syndrome. If all of the long bones are short, this may indicate a form of dwarfism.

- o **Thickened nuchal fold** is the skin fold in the back of the fetal neck. This finding increases the risk for Down syndrome and cardiac abnormalities.

- o **Nasal bone not present** may be an indication of Down syndrome or another chromosomal abnormality.

- o **Two-vessel cord** is seen in about 1 percent of fetuses. The two-vessel cord can be a sign of other fetal birth defects, so a level 2 ultrasound scan should be performed. Genetic counseling should also be offered. Over 50 percent of two-vessel cords occur because the third vessel collapses early in the pregnancy. There is no increased risk to the fetus because of this finding.

If your ultrasound has detected the presence of one of more soft markers, you will likely be referred to a high-risk specialist. At this point, you should already have your nuchal translucency/PAPP-A results and possibly your quad screen results, which will have given you a risk figure for having a baby with a chromosomal abnormality. If you are *under* the age of 35 and there is one soft marker present, your risk will rise slightly, but usually not enough to place you in a high-risk category. However, if you are *over* the age of 35 and have one soft marker present, you will then be placed in a high-risk category, even if your screening-test results showed your risk as being low. You will then be counseled for diagnostic testing.

Regardless of your age, if an ultrasound detects *two or more* soft markers, you are automatically placed in a high-risk category for having a baby with a chromosomal abnormality and will be counseled for diagnostic testing.

Ultrasound-Detailed (Level 2)
This is usually performed 18–22 weeks of gestation at radiology centers or perinatal centers by high-risk, maternal-fetal specialists with special training in detecting birth defects. A detailed level 2 study looks at the fetal head anatomy, face, hands, arms, neck, chest, heart, spine, kidneys, stomach, bladder, sex organs, placenta, cord insertion (baby and placenta), legs, feet, membranes, and the mother's cervix. Detailed ultrasounds can be used to diagnose structural abnormalities of the fetus.

Many centers now have 3D ultrasound technology. This technology makes it much easier for a birth defect to be diagnosed that might not have been easily seen on a standard 2D ultrasound image.

Many patients are never offered a detailed level 2 ultrasound unless their previous ultrasound or blood work put them into a high-risk category. It is important to note that 70 percent of babies with birth defects are found in the younger, low-risk population. If you want this type of ultrasound, you often have to request it.

Limits to Ultrasound
You should be aware of the limitations of prenatal ultrasound for the detection of chromosomal abnormalities. Up to 50 percent of babies with a chromosomal abnormality have normal ultrasound findings, which means the baby looks completely normal by ultrasound. When looking for signs of a chromosomal abnormality, ultrasound is just a screening tool and can never completely rule out this kind of abnormality. An ultrasound examination can be limited in its ability, to a lesser or greater degree, depending on a variety of factors ranging from gestational age to the competence of the technician performing it.

Limits to ultrasound effectiveness can be due to:
- Gestational age
- Fetal position
- Multiple gestation
- Maternal obesity
- Prior abdominal surgery
- Knowledge and experience of the technician performing the exam

 Diagnostic Testing

Prenatal diagnostic tests are invasive tests that examine fetal cells and actually diagnose chromosomal abnormalities or other specific conditions affecting the fetus. These prenatal diagnostic tests are 99.9 percent accurate. If your screening tests are negative, you can always request that a diagnostic test be performed.

The diagnostic tests that you may be offered during your pregnancy include:

Chorionic Villus Sampling (CVS)

CVS is an invasive procedure that is performed at 10½–13 weeks' gestation by a maternal-fetal medicine specialist. This procedure is performed either abdominally or vaginally by ultrasound guidance. The test samples the placenta, which contains fetal DNA. It should be noted that CVS cannot be used to diagnose neural tube defects.

Amniocentesis

Amniocentesis is an invasive procedure that is performed at 15–22 weeks' gestation by an ob/gyn or maternal-fetal medicine specialist. This procedure is performed abdominally by ultrasound guidance. The test samples the amniotic fluid, which contains fetal cells, for analysis.

Amniocentesis can additionally be recommended during the third trimester to test fetal lung maturity before week 38. This is most commonly done when the doctor is considering an earlier delivery because of gestational diabetes.

Although amniocentesis and CVS can detect greater than 99 percent of the identifiable chromosomal abnormalities, and amniocentesis can detect 98 percent of neural tube defects, there still is no guarantee that you will have a perfectly normal baby. These diagnostic tests cannot detect all causes of birth defects, genetic diseases, or mental retardation.

Percutaneous Umbilical Cord Blood Sampling (PUBS)

A PUBS is performed at 16–40 weeks' gestation by insertion of a needle into the umbilical vein, near the placenta, under ultrasound guidance. This test is done if it is necessary to analyze fetal cells for diagnosis or evaluation of certain medical conditions affecting the fetus. This procedure is done very infrequently.

CHAPTER 23

More on Amniocentesis and Chorionic Villus Sampling (CVS)

It used to be that only women aged 35 and older were offered diagnostic testing. It is now recommended that all women be offered the option of having an amniocentesis or CVS regardless of their age.

The following information should address most of your concerns regarding these types of procedures.

Isn't it true that only women over 35 need diagnostic testing?

Women of any age can have a baby with a chromosomal abnormality or birth defect.

If the screening tests are normal, do I need to worry about Down syndrome?

If you have a screening result showing a very low risk, such as one in 2,500 or one in 5,000, you must understand that the baby can still have a chromosomal abnormality. Often, if the risk is low, you will be told the result is "normal" or "negative." Many couples take this to mean that the baby has no chance of having these problems. This is not true.

In the medical profession of obstetrics, we would not

recommend an amniocentesis or CVS for these low screening results. This is because the risk of loss from the testing itself is greater than the chance of the baby having a chromosomal abnormality.

However, if you and your partner want a yes-or-no answer as to whether the baby has Down syndrome or other chromosomal abnormalities, then you *must* have an amniocentesis or CVS.

Is the risk of having a miscarriage high after an amniocentesis or CVS?

Not if you have the procedure performed by a physician who does several hundred per year. The risk for any complications at perinatal centers resulting from having an amniocentesis is usually no higher than one in 1,600. The complication rate after a CVS is about one in 300. The miscarriage rate for CVS is higher than for amniocentesis, not due to the procedure itself, but due to the fact that it is done at the end of the first trimester when the risk of spontaneous abortion is greater. Post-procedure instructions must be followed in order to keep your risk low.

How is an amniocentesis done?

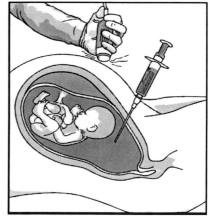

The procedure is done at 15–22 weeks of gestation and can be done in your doctor's office. Before the procedure begins, an ultrasound will be preformed to determine the baby's position. The doctor will then decide on a location to obtain a sample of amniotic fluid that surrounds the baby. Your belly will be cleaned with an antiseptic solution before the procedure begins. Using continuous ultrasound guidance, a very thin needle is inserted through your abdomen to collect a half ounce of amniotic fluid in the attached syringe. After the fluid has been collected, the needle is removed, the baby's heart rate is calculated, and the mom is helped off the ultrasound table. The procedure itself takes about two minutes to perform.

☝ How is a CVS performed?

A CVS is done at 10 ½–13 weeks' gestation. If you are having a transabdominal CVS, the same procedure will be followed as in an amniocentesis, except that placental tissue will be obtained instead of amniotic fluid. The procedure takes about three minutes to perform.

If you are having a transcervical CVS, you will lie on your back and put your feet in stirrups. Your vaginal area will be cleaned with an antiseptic solution, and a small catheter will be placed into your vagina through your cervix and into the placenta. A syringe will be attached to the catheter, and suction will be applied to withdraw a small amount of placental tissue. This procedure is also performed under continuous ultrasound guidance.

☝ Does having an amniocentesis or CVS hurt?

One of the biggest misconceptions about amniocentesis and CVS is that the procedure is painful. Having the procedure is very much like having your blood drawn, except the needle that is used during this testing is much thinner. If you stay relaxed during the procedure and do not tense your stomach muscles, you will only feel a small stick when the needle first enters your skin.

A transcervical CVS feels very much like a Pap smear examination. You might experience some mild cramping afterward.

⁇ Are there any special instructions for after an amniocentesis or CVS is done?

All women having these procedures should rest for 24 hours and protect their abdominal area from injury. This includes:

o No lifting

o No wearing tight belts

o No standing for any significant amount of time

If there is a chance that a child or pet can jump on your belly while you are lying down, put a pillow over your belly to stay protected. Having cramps or light vaginal spotting is common for both procedures 5–10 percent of the time. If you experience a gush of clear fluid after an amniocentesis, with or without cramping, you should get in touch with the doctor who did the procedure. A pregnancy complication occurring one week following diagnostic testing should not be attributed to the procedure.

⁇ How long does it take to get the results?

Results are usually available in 7–10 days. This can vary by up to one week or more if the cells from the amniocentesis or CVS are slow to grow in the lab. This can be caused by many outside factors and does not mean there is something wrong with the baby.

There is also a method called *fluorescence in situ hybridization* (FISH) that can provide a rapid preliminary result within 48 hours for the most common chromosomal abnormalities (Trisomy 13, 18, and 21, and problems with the X or Y chromosome). The results are not final until all the chromosomes have been analyzed.

Why would a woman choose to have a CVS instead of an amniocentesis?

Women who are of advanced maternal age (35 or over) have a higher risk for chromosomal abnormalities (or who just want to know very early in their pregnancy) will have a CVS to get this information in the first trimester of pregnancy, instead of an amniocentesis. However, if you have a family history of neural tube defects or have already had a child with a neural tube defect, you will need to have an amniocentesis, as a CVS cannot be used to test for this condition.

Is it true that CVS can cause birth defects?

About 20 years ago, a few medical centers in the United States and Europe started to investigate whether CVS could be performed between eight and 10 weeks' gestation. Because all the major organ systems and long bones of the fetus were not yet completely formed, a higher incidence of limb defects was seen. This was most likely due to a disruption of blood flow from the placenta when the procedure was done. When CVS was performed after 10½ weeks, studies concluded that there was no greater risk of having a baby with a limb defect than among the general population that did not have CVS.

What if my risk is low and my insurance will not pay for diagnostic testing?

Many insurance companies will only pay for diagnostic testing if you are over 35 or there is a medical suspicion that an abnormality is present. Check with your insurance company to see whether a routine amniocentesis or CVS is covered on your policy.

I am a person who would never end a pregnancy, even if there were a problem. Why should I even think about having an amniocentesis or CVS?

Women often ask this question in the course of a discussion about birth defect detection. If you are at a higher risk for having a baby with a chromosomal or genetic abnormality, your baby could need special newborn care. Should the baby be found to have a birth defect that a level I or II hospital cannot handle, the baby may have to be transferred to a level III center. Knowing the results of diagnostic testing will allow you to arrange to deliver your baby at a level III medical center that has a neonatal, special-care nursery. This has nothing to do with interrupting the pregnancy, but would allow you to prepare for any problems that may arise and decide on the correct type of hospital to use for delivery.

CHAPTER 24

When a Birth Defect Is Found

Bringing a child into the world is usually a time filled with much joy and excitement. The last thing an expectant mother expects to hear is that her unborn baby has been diagnosed with a birth defect.

News of a problem always seems unreal. In an instant, all your hopes and dreams for this new baby now seem uncertain. Even though you have never met this little person, you already love him or her and have a broken heart, knowing your baby might have a difficult life ahead. It is common to feel a loss of the perfect baby you were expecting.

It is important to gather as much information as possible so that you and your partner can make an informed choice as to how you want to proceed with the pregnancy.

 ## Questions for Your Doctor:

- Are there other physicians who might be able to give us more information about this type of abnormality or condition?

- Are there any associated health conditions related to the abnormality my baby was diagnosed with?

- What are the chances that the tests are incorrect?

- ○ Will the baby survive?
- ○ What type of special care will this child need?
- ○ Are there support groups in the area that deal with children who have this condition?
- ○ Is there another doctor I can get a second opinion from?
- ○ What are the chances this will happen again in another pregnancy?

Even though it may be easier said than done, it is important to try to stay calm during this very difficult time. It is common to go into denial and not accept what is really happening. Many moms feel they did something to cause this, but the truth is that nothing could have been done to prevent it.

It is important for you and your partner to be there for each other through this period. Try to come to a decision together as to whether you are going to continue the pregnancy or interrupt it. Your doctor will likely help you through this time and answer any questions that you have.

Remember that when a problem like this happens, the information is private and you should not feel obligated to tell family or friends unless you want to. Counseling is often a good idea to help you through the emotions and come to a place of peace with whatever decisions you need to make for your baby and yourself.

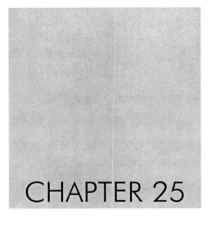

CHAPTER 25

Pre-delivery Antenatal Testing for Pregnancy Complications

Checking the well-being or good health of your baby during the last one to two months of your pregnancy is a common practice in modern obstetrics. This is done if there is any need to check the health of the fetus, but not all women need this type of testing.

These tests include ultrasound, fetal heart rate monitoring, and detection of blood flow to the baby from the placenta. This testing cannot correct a problem, but can let you and your doctor know if you need closer monitoring or need to plan for a possible early delivery before you go into labor.

 ## Typical Reasons for Antenatal Fetal Evaluation

- Hypertension
- Gestational diabetes
- Type 2 diabetes
- Small fetus
- Illicit drug use
- Smoking
- Chronic medical illnesses

- Advanced maternal age (over 35)
- Multiple gestation
- Oligohydramnios (insufficient fluid)
- Polyhydramnios (excess fluid)
- Unexplained high AFP values
- Second/third trimester bleeding
- History of a stillbirth
- IVF (in vitro fertilization) pregnancy
- Trauma during the pregnancy
- Diagnosed birth defect
- Fetal cardiac problems (rhythm problem or diagnosis of abnormal heart)
- Severe asthma
- Autoimmune disorders
- Rh incompatibility
- Morbid obesity (BMI >35)
- Maternal heart disease
- Preeclampsia
- Post-date pregnancy (41 weeks and beyond)
- Preterm labor
- Ruptured membranes

Pre-Delivery Antenatal Tests for Complicated Pregnancies

- **NST (non-stress test):** monitors the fetal heart and looks for good variable heartbeat minute by minute. A fetal heartbeat that remains the same over many minutes can mean that the baby is sleeping or that the baby is not getting an adequate amount of oxygen for a change in the heart rate. If you have a non-reactive non-stress test, further antenatal testing should be performed *that day* to confirm the baby's well-being.

○ **BPP (biophysical profile):** an ultrasound evaluation of the fluid surrounding the baby, fetal movement, and fetal breathing motion. This is a better test than NST because it provides more information to the doctors about the baby's health in the womb.

○ **Doppler evaluation:** measures blood flow from the placenta to the baby, and gives information to your doctor concerning the baby's health as it relates to oxygen and nutrition supply.

○ **VAS (vibroacoustic stimulation):** a modification of the NST, this testing uses a vibrating instrument on the mom's abdomen to determine the fetus's response to sound. This can be added to the NST to wake up a sleeping baby.

In general, a baby with normal fetal testing has a better than 99 percent chance of doing well inside the womb for the next seven days, or until the next weekly testing session, as described above. If the antenatal testing indicates a problem, then the testing can be repeated the following day, or in some cases, the baby may need to be delivered early.

In conclusion, good weekly antenatal testing gives the mom and her obstetrician reassurance that the pregnancy can continue for at least one more week. So try to relax between visits!

 ## Post-Date Pregnancy

I'll bet you did not know that only 3 out of 100 women deliver on their due date. The majority of women deliver within one week of that date. Between seven days before and seven days after the due date is when the majority of women will deliver.

If you go more than seven days beyond your due date, you will be in the post-date pregnancy period. From that point on, for 7–10 days, you should have antenatal testing to make certain the baby is active and there is an adequate amount of amniotic fluid surrounding it. For many years, the medical community felt that a pregnancy could safely go to 43 weeks before a woman should be delivered. However, this year, a multi-center study showed that a baby in the womb beyond 41 completed weeks begins to have an increased risk for newborn problems.

Talk with your doctor about how far you will be permitted to go beyond your due date before you are delivered.

 ## Kick Counts

Kick counts have been used during pregnancy for many years. They are used to access fetal well-being by the mom-to-be.

Starting in the third trimester, you should start paying attention to your baby's kicking patterns. The best time to do this is when you are relaxing after a meal. The general recommendation is that you should feel your baby kick 10 times in a one- to two- hour period. This may occur during the first 30 minutes, and then you can discontinue counting. If 10 kicks are not felt within two hours, you should repeat this test in the next few hours. If a second kick count does not produce 10 kicks in one to two hours, you should contact your healthcare provider.

After 36 weeks, it is normal to have fewer kicks and more rolling motions of the baby due to restricted space. Rolling motions would be counted as a kick during your kick count.

 ## Conditions that make kick-counting especially important:

- ○ Diabetes
- ○ Hypertension
- ○ Current preterm labor

o Fetal growth restriction

o Oligohydramnios (low amniotic fluid)

Performing kick counts during pregnancy is an important function to access fetal well-being, but also gives the mom-to-be a chance to bond with her baby while it is still inside of her.

CHAPTER 26

Fetal Ultrasound Evaluations for Growth

In the late second trimester and throughout the third trimester, your doctor may have you get an ultrasound if the baby is thought to be either smaller or larger than your dates would indicate.

The most accurate ultrasound for dating your pregnancy is in the first trimester between week six and week 12. This is because everyone's fetus is the same size in the first trimester. So, a fetal measurement at eight to nine weeks' gestation in Denver, Colorado, is the same as an eight-to-nine-week fetus in London, England. However, as you go further into the second trimester and through the third trimester, everyone's fetus measures either a little larger or smaller than the average-size fetus. A 32-week fetus can weigh anywhere between three and five pounds, depending on many factors including family genetics for newborn size.

 ### Facts about Ultrasound Evaluations Used for Determining Fetal Size

o   If you had an early ultrasound, the date determined then is always your due date.

o   The ultrasound looking for size never changes your due date, whether yours is a larger or a smaller fetus. The ultrasound may say that your baby measures the size of a fetus at 36 weeks' gestation, but you thought you were really at 33 weeks (based on your LMP and early scan). This means your fetus is three weeks ahead of the average-size 33-week fetus, not that you are now 36 weeks along and due three weeks sooner.

o   Fetal size can run between the 1st percentile and 99th percentile. This means that a fetus in the 1st percentile is very small, and 99 out of 100 babies are larger than your baby at its gestational age. A baby in the 50th percentile is right in the middle, meaning 50 percent of fetuses are smaller than this baby, and 50 percent are larger.

o   Estimates of fetal size in the third trimester are not accurate and can range three-quarters of a pound either way from the estimated weight.

CHAPTER 27

Congenital Birth Defects Most Often Seen

A defect that is present at birth is called a congenital birth defect. The vast majority of these defects are random occurrences and cannot be prevented. About 1 in 50 babies are born with a mild to severe birth defect. The birth defects listed below are the most common that can be seen by ultrasound. Frequently, these defects can be corrected following birth.

 ## Cardiac Abnormalities

Structural heart abnormalities, which can range from very mild to very serious, are the most common congenital abnormalities found in newborn babies, occurring in 1 in 130 live-born infants. The most common heart defects that are seen are usually mild and do not require any type of surgery. Those that do need surgery have a much better prognosis today than they did just 10 years ago.

A close evaluation of the fetal heart during a level 2 ultrasound at 18–20 weeks is extremely important, and all women who are carrying a fetus with a heart abnormality should have an amniocentesis. Nearly 20 percent of all babies with a heart abnormality have a chromosomal abnormality. Level 1 anatomy scans can only identify 10–20 percent of fetal heart defects, while a detailed level 2 study picks up 80 percent of congenital heart defects.

Young pregnant women with no risk factors are as much at risk for a fetal heart defect as are older pregnant women. This is why it is very important for all pregnant women to have an anatomy ultrasound (level 2) between 18 and 20 weeks' gestation. Over 70 percent of all babies born with birth defects are born to low-risk, young women.

Any baby with a congenital heart defect should be delivered at a level III medical center with a Neonatal Intensive Care Unit (NICU).

 ## Gastroschisis

Gastroschisis is a birth defect where parts of the fetal bowel loop outside of the body, free-floating in the amniotic fluid. This abnormality occurs in approximately 1 in 1,000 live births. The bowel comes out at the insertion site of the umbilical cord. This condition is more often seen in babies of younger women. These defects are usually isolated, and less than 1 percent have any associated problems, but an amniocentesis is still strongly recommended to get the pediatric team all this information for the birth. The bowel is placed back into the baby by a pediatric surgeon after birth. The majority of these babies do very well after surgery.

There is no reason why the baby cannot be delivered vaginally, but most of the time a C-section is performed.

 ## Renal Abnormalities

Kidney abnormalities are usually identified at the 20-week ultrasound evaluation. This is seen in about 1 in 400 fetuses. Severe renal disease is usually accompanied by low amniotic fluid surrounding the fetus (oligohydramnios). This is because, with severe kidney disease, the fetal kidneys produce very little urine, and amniotic fluid is fetal urine. Without fetal urine (amniotic fluid), the fetal lungs do not develop, and the fetus cannot breathe after birth. These babies either require renal surgery or do not survive the newborn period. If a baby does not have kidneys, this is called renal agenesis or Potters syndrome, and is more common in boys. These babies cannot survive after birth.

 ## Hydronephrosis

This condition features enlarged kidneys and is seen in 1 in 50 fetuses, more commonly in males. Excess fluid is often due to a narrowing or blockage of the ureters, which are the tubes connecting the kidneys to the bladder. This can be a marker for chromosomal abnormality, and you should be counseled for a possible amniocentesis. The hydronephrosis by itself is not a serious problem and can often correct itself after birth. Your pediatrician may send you to a pediatric renal specialist in the first few months following birth.

 ## Cleft Lip and Palate

Cleft lip and palate occur when the upper lip and lower lip fail to join (fuse) correctly in the eighth to ninth week of pregnancy. This can occur on one side of the face, or both. Nearly 60 syndromes or other groups of birth defects can be associated with cleft lip and palate. A detailed, high-level ultrasound should be performed by a maternal-fetal medicine specialist to make certain there are no other detectable birth defects, and an amniocentesis should be discussed with your doctor.

This abnormality happens in about 1 in every 300–400 live births. If cleft lip/palate runs in the family of the mother or father, there is a 1 in 25 risk of it happening in their future children. Surgery is available to correct this condition, and the prognosis is excellent.

Clubfoot

A clubfoot is a common birth defect occurring in about 1 in 1,000 live births. About 50 percent occur in both feet, and are twice as common in males.

The most common cause is idiopathic, meaning unknown. Clubfoot does run in families and there is a 2–3 percent chance of passing down clubfoot from one of the parents (usually Dad) to the children. Genetic birth defects (Trisomy 18 or Edwards syndrome) are associated with clubfoot. Limb and skeletal abnormalities and several other syndromes totaling over 25 can be associated with clubfoot. Clubfoot can be seen as early as 15–18 weeks with ultrasound during the pregnancy. Treatment includes manipulation, surgery, casting, and wrapping the ankle and foot, depending on the specific child.

 ## Omphalocele

Omphalocele is a problem occurring only in about 1 in 5,000 live births. This is an abdominal wall defect where portions of the bowel and liver are outside of the body, covered by the peritoneal membrane. Nearly 50 percent of these children have chromosomal abnormalities. Babies with this condition often have cardiac abnormalities, and close to 40 percent do not survive the newborn period. An amniocentesis and fetal echocardiogram are recommended with this diagnosis. Surgery can be performed, but depending on the specific case, it may or may not be successful.

CHAPTER 28

Down Syndrome

I first learned about Down syndrome in 1974 when I was getting my degree in genetic counseling in New Jersey. For the past 35 years, I have worked with hundreds of parents who have had an increased risk of passing on a chromosome problem (such as Down syndrome) to a child or had a diagnosis of a chromosomal disorder.

Down syndrome, also known as Down's, as well as Trisomy 21, is the most commonly occurring chromosome abnormality seen in pregnant women. While Down syndrome occurs more frequently in older women, 70 percent of all children with Down syndrome are born to women under the age of 35 years. This is because more women under the age of 35 are having children.

Down syndrome occurs in about 1 in 800 live births. Currently, more than 400,000 people are living with this syndrome in the United States.

? What causes Down Syndrome?

Over 99 percent of the time, the incidence of Down syndrome is due to a random event that occurs during cell division shortly after fertilization. A person normally has 46 chromosomes, 23 inherited from each parent. Down syndrome is caused when a person has three copies of chromosome 21 instead of two copies.

Conception in a **woman over the age of 35 or by a man over the age of 50 will increase the risk of this occurring.** About 1–2 percent of the time, there is a variation in the chromosomes of one of the parents, called a *Robertsonian translocation,* that results in a higher risk of a child being born with Down syndrome. It is not caused by any behavioral activity of either parent or by any environmental factors. Down syndrome only runs in families with these Robertsonian translocations and cannot be prevented.

❓ Can my doctor tell me whether my child will be mildly or severely affected?

No. It usually takes several years before everyone will know the potential of your child. Down syndrome affects each child's ability to learn in different ways, but most will have mild to moderate intellectual impairment.

❓ What types of health problems do children with Down syndrome have?

While some children with Down syndrome have no significant health problems, others may experience many medical issues that require extra care. Almost half of all children born with Down's will have congenital heart defects. They are also at an increased risk of developing pulmonary hypertension. Nearly half of all children with Down's will have hearing and vision problems. Children with Down's may also suffer from thyroid problems, intestinal abnormalities, an increased susceptibility to infection, seizure disorder, and respiratory problems.

❓ Why has the incidence of Down syndrome increased in the United States?

More children are being born with Down syndrome than were 10 years ago. There are a few reasons why this is occurring.

- ○ More women over the age of 35 are having children.
- ○ More women are relying on screening tests that are "negative" and not having diagnostic testing.
- ○ More women are getting pregnant through IVF and will not have any invasive testing performed if they believe their risk of miscarriage would increase.
- ○ More women are choosing to keep a baby with Down syndrome after a diagnosis is made.

If you have received news that your unborn baby has been diagnosed with Down syndrome, you will probably be overwhelmed with many emotions, especially fear of the unknown. It is important to get as much information and support as you need. Your doctor may be able to put you in touch with other mothers who have had children with Down syndrome or may be able to direct you to a local support group.

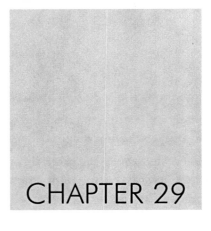

CHAPTER 29

Neural Tube Defects and Other Neurological Abnormalities

These birth defects comprise some of the most common and serious congenital abnormalities that we can detect in the early prenatal period. In the absence of any screening, nearly 1 in 400 babies are born with some form of spinal abnormality.

 ## Spina Bifida

Spina bifida has several variations. The most common type of spina bifida is where there is an open area of the spine in the lower back. This is called a myelomeningocele and often results in mild to severe mental retardation and varying degrees of physical handicaps, which can include difficulty walking, inability to control urination and bowel control. Recurrence is higher for birth mothers who have had a previous child with spina bifida. Genetic counseling is strongly recommended for couples in this situation.

The most severe form of spina bifida is anencephaly, in which the skull bones (cranium) do not completely form, and the brain is underdeveloped. These infants die either in the womb or shortly after birth.

The mildest form of spinal abnormality is spina bifida occulta, which affects 5 percent of all live-born children. Spina bifida occulta is a malformed spinal cord closure that does not cause paralysis or require surgery. This abnormality usually goes unnoticed and causes few problems throughout the life of the affected individual.

A blood (serum) screening for maternal serum AFP (alpha-fetoprotein) taken at 16–20 weeks' gestation, as well as an advanced anatomy ultrasound, can help diagnose myelomeningocele and anencephaly in your unborn child. However, the only definite diagnosis of spina bifida can come from an amniocentesis, which can detect the presence of acetylcholinesterase (AChE) in the amniotic fluid. Acetylcholinesterase, an enzyme in fetal spinal fluid, should not be present in the amniotic fluid. When it is, the fetus is likely to have spina bifida. The only other reason AChE would be present is if the baby has an abdominal wall defect like gastroschisis.

The incidence of spina bifida can be reduced by 75 percent if folic acid is taken three months prior to conception and throughout the first trimester. Taking 400–800 micrograms is needed.

 ## Hydrocephalus

There are many abnormalities that can result in excessive fluid collections in the fetal head that may result in hydrocephalus (enlarged fetal head) or enlarged ventricles (fluid-filled areas of the brain). The finding of excessive fluid in the head can be attributed to chromosomal abnormalities, anatomical defects, or environmental causes. Half of the time, a cause cannot be determined. The results of excessive fluid vary from no effect (a completely normal outcome) to mild, moderate, or severe mental retardation. One out of four babies with hydrocephalus does not survive the first year of life.

A fetus with this diagnosis should be evaluated by a high-risk obstetrician. Further tests can be performed to more clearly determine the possible cause of the excessive fluid. The use of MRI (magnetic resonance imaging) or CT scanning may be helpful in determining a cause. The couple should seek counseling with a specialist to explore possible outcomes.

 ## Cerebral Palsy

Cerebral palsy is a muscular and neurologic motor disorder involving one or more limbs that can result in muscular spasticity or paralysis. Both epilepsy and mental retardation can also be associated with cerebral palsy.

For over 140 years, doctors have been describing the symptoms of cerebral palsy and debating what causes it. Today, most researchers believe there is an association of periods of decreased oxygen during the pregnancy that lead to an increased risk of cerebral palsy. These periods of decreased oxygen are thought to be related to multiple gestations, placenta complications, the age of the mother, and cigarette smoking.

After delivery, your physician or midwife can request a test of the fetal blood gas obtained from the umbilical cord. This test will determine if the baby had a dangerously low level of oxygen just prior to delivery. If this is the case, the pediatrician should be made aware of this finding for use during the baby's newborn evaluation. A normal blood gas just after birth, combined with signs of neurologic damage, would suggest a period of low oxygen to the fetus sometime during the pregnancy and not during the labor and delivery period.

Despite the dramatic increase in cesarean sections (25 percent of all deliveries), the percentage of children affected with cerebral palsy has not decreased. It occurs in approximately 1 in every 500 live births. This risk has not changed over the last 60 years. In fact, the numbers have increased slightly because preterm babies now have a better chance of survival, and preterm babies are more likely to be affected with cerebral palsy.

There is very little that a mother can do to reduce this risk of cerebral palsy. Certainly for a mother to be in good health by getting her weight in good control, as well as keeping her blood pressure and/or diabetes in check, will be of benefit. In addition, giving up cigarette smoking cuts the risk of cerebral palsy.

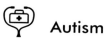 ## Autism

Autism is a neurological disorder that can result in a child's inability to learn language and relate to other people.

I have had expectant moms ask me if I could tell if their child had autism during an ultrasound examination. Unfortunately, a diagnosis usually does not occur until one to three years of life; it cannot be diagnosed before birth.

It is now felt that autism may be caused by many different factors, including genetics, the environment, and perhaps vaccinations. Extensive research is currently ongoing to look for early diagnosis and treatment protocols.

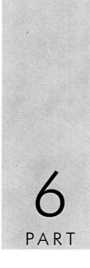

6

PART

MATERNAL MEDICAL COMPLICATIONS

CHAPTER 30

Obesity Risks and Pregnancy

As I have said elsewhere in this book, the best gift you can give your baby-to-be or soon-to-be-conceived child is a healthy mother. Obesity is the most pressing and serious issue in our country. Medical illnesses affect you more seriously when you are 40–50 pounds overweight. This means you should not weigh more than 20 percent above the ideal weight for your age and height.

Second only to smoking, obesity causes tremendous risks to both the mother and baby during and after a pregnancy (see table 30.1). Babies born to obese women have a higher risk of being in the NICU (neonatal intensive care unit). They are also at a much higher risk of being born with a birth defect. The risk of neural tube defects (spina bifida) are double that of a woman of normal weight. *Extra folic acid may not protect a pregnant woman who is obese from having a baby with spina bifida.*

Maternal obesity can cause many obstacles when it comes to trying to get a good view of your baby's anatomy through ultrasound. Unfortunately, many times a doctor cannot reassure a woman that everything looks fine with the baby. This is especially true when it comes to the fetal heart and craniospinal structures. Because visualization tends to be very poor in obese patients, it is important to consider having an amniocentesis, which would rule out neural tube defects and most chromosomal abnormalities.

Table 30.1: Pregnancy Complication
Risks Associated With Obesity

Preeclampsia	4–5 times higher
Stillbirth	3–4 times higher
C-section	2–3 times higher
Gestational diabetes	4–5 times higher
Early newborn death	2–3 times higher
Hypertension	4–5 times higher
Infertility	4–5 times higher
Cost of pregnancy/delivery	6–8 times higher

Any woman who is overweight and thinking about getting pregnant needs a complete physical by her doctor. An evaluation should be done for hypertension, diabetes, and thyroid disorders.

In addition, any woman who is overweight should work on getting her weight in better control before getting pregnant. If you have had a weight issue for a long time, then you should see a weight-control specialist or nutritionist who may suggest a special weight-loss plan for you.

You should not go on a diet thinking that once you have lost some weight you can get pregnant and start eating like you used to. You should change the way you eat to a balanced plan, such as one recommended by Weight Watchers, and stay on that healthy plan for at least six months prior to getting pregnant. Even if you lose only 15–30 pounds before you conceive, that is still a great start to a healthier pregnancy and a healthier lifestyle.

 ## Complication Risks Associated with Delivery

Many women who are obese will have difficulty in achieving a vaginal birth. Between 40 and 50 percent will need a C-section. The most common reasons are the baby being particularly large or the mother having difficulty getting through the second stage of labor.

Women who are heavy, with a BMI over 30 or a weight greater than 250 pounds, and need a C-section should discuss with their doctor the location on the abdomen where the incision will be made. The majority of women have a low, transverse incision (side to side) above the pubic hair-line. However, heavy women can have great difficulty with this type of incision. When the skin incision is covered by the belly, it raises the risk of infection and prolongs healing.

It is recommended by the American College of Obstetrics and Gynecology (ACOG) that a transverse incision be made on obese women two to three inches below the belly button. This permits healing and allows the mother to see and care for the incision herself. I have made several hundred of these incisions with excellent outcomes.

CHAPTER 31

Becoming Pregnant after Gastric Surgery

Many women today are having gastric bypass or lap-band surgeries performed before becoming pregnant. Most women with this surgery do well during their pregnancy, but there is an optimal waiting period for each of these to ensure a healthy mother and baby.

Doctors recommend that you wait 18 months after gastric bypass surgery before becoming pregnant because this is the period when rapid weight loss is occurring. Such rapid weight loss may deprive a developing baby of the nutrients it needs to grow.

Lap-band surgery produces a more gradual weight loss and does not cause such nutritional problems. You should still wait at least six months before getting pregnant so that you have time to get to a healthier weight.

It is important that all women who have had gastric surgery meet with their internist or gastrointestinal specialist to go over any special dietary recommendations that should be followed during the pregnancy. A restricted calorie diet will not place a pregnancy at risk as long as the mom does not have *malabsorption syndrome,* which causes a loss of vitamins and necessary nutrition from the food she eats.

If nausea and vomiting complicate the pregnancy for

any reason, the use of medications and supplemental fluids, protein drinks, B-complex vitamins, and even IV fluids may be necessary. Working with a nutritionist or dietician during the entire pregnancy may be something to consider.

CHAPTER 32

Antiphospholipid Antibody Syndrome and Blood Clotting Disorders in Pregnancy

Women with a history of blood clots, multiple pregnancy losses, or stillbirths need to be tested for a certain type of cell protein antibody that can cause blood clots in the legs and lungs. These disorders can be both inherited or occur in women spontaneously. This often occurs after one or two normal pregnancies followed by multiple miscarriages. All of these antibodies we are speaking of will slowly destroy the placenta with micro-blood clots in the first, second, or third trimester. This can seriously put your health, your baby's health, and your pregnancy at risk.

 ## Inherited Abnormalities that Cause Blood Clotting

- ○ MTHFR (methylenetetrahydrofolate reductase)
- ○ Factor V Leiden
- ○ Protein C deficiency
- ○ Protein S deficiency
- ○ Anti-thrombin III deficiency
- ○ Anticardiolipin antibodies
- ○ Lupus anticoagulant

Pregnancy Risks Associated with Antiphospholipid Syndrome

- Multiple pregnancy losses
- Blood clots (10–25 percent in mothers not treated)
- Preeclampsia (30–40 percent)
- Fetal growth problems (small baby)
- Preterm delivery
- Stillbirth
- Anemia
- Lupus
- Low platelet count (clotting)
- Higher C-section rate

Treatments for Blood-Clotting Disorders

- Take baby aspirin (81 mg) once daily starting the month that you begin attempting to get pregnant.
- Wear graduated compression stockings (thigh high).
- Receive low-dose and low-molecular-weight heparin, given by injection, once or twice a day. Your doctor will discuss this with you.
- Close evaluation of the fetus, with multiple growth studies and antenatal testing (biophysical profiles, Doppler studies), should be done weekly from 34 weeks till delivery.
- Delivery should take place by inducing labor or C-section if you're not delivered by 38 completed weeks of gestation.

Your own obstetrician may alter these recommendations depending on specific factors that are unique to you.

If you are diagnosed with a blood-clotting disorder and are not treated with aspirin and/or heparin, your risk of early delivery or pregnancy loss will be 80 percent, leaving only a 20 percent chance of having a successful pregnancy. If you are treated, the statistics are reversed, with an 80 percent chance of a successful outcome.

CHAPTER 33

Women with Heart Disease Who Are Pregnant

Pregnancy puts significant stress on your heart and your circulatory system. During your first trimester, there is an increase in the stress placed on the cardiac muscle. This increases significantly in the second and third trimesters, as well as during labor and delivery. There is again major stress on the heart just following delivery. If you have a history of heart disease, I cannot stress enough the importance of having a complete cardiac evaluation with an EKG or an echocardiogram, if appropriate. Should medications be involved, I suggest seeing a high-risk obstetrician to discuss any and all potential risks that heart medications could have on your pregnancy.

Women who were born with congenital heart disease have a 2–3 percent risk of giving birth to a child with a heart problem. While low, this is four to five times greater than the general population's risk. All women with a history of congenital heart disease should have a *fetal echocardiogram* 18–22 weeks into their pregnancy.

 ### Conditions that Increase the Risk of Fetal Congenital Heart Disease

○ History of congenital heart disease in the family

- Chronic high blood pressure
- Diabetes (type I or II)
- Morbid obesity
- Uncontrolled thyroid disease
- Smoking
- Drug abuse
- Previous child with congenital heart disease

Anemia is a serious concern for any woman who has a history of cardiac disease. If this describes your situation, you should take additional iron throughout your pregnancy to get your blood count (hemoglobin) higher so that anemia does not worsen your heart disease.

Because blood infections are fairly common during labor and delivery, the use of antibiotics is common for women with cardiac disease. Blood-thinning drugs are sometimes used during the pregnancy as well, varying from patient to patient.

CHAPTER 34

Pregnancy and Thyroid Disease

Thyroid diseases are the second most common endocrine disorder that affects women of reproductive age. If you know you have a thyroid condition, you should see your internist or treating physician prior to getting pregnant to make sure your thyroid levels are within normal range. Make sure that your ob/gyn is aware that you are being treated for this condition.

Occasionally, thyroid disease does not show signs or symptoms until a woman becomes pregnant.

 ## Hyperthyroidism (Overactive Thyroid)

This occurs in about 1 in 500 pregnant women. The most common cause of excessive thyroid production is Graves' disease. Symptoms of an overactive thyroid include a rapid heartbeat, tremors, nervousness, excessive sweating, and frequent bowel movements. Symptoms tend to be worse in the first half of the pregnancy and to lessen during the second half, recurring after the baby is born.

Hyperthyroidism in pregnancy is usually treated with PTU (propylthiouracil). This medication is considered safe for use during pregnancy at its *lowest recommended dose*. If left untreated, there is a greater risk of preterm delivery, severe preeclampsia, a low-birth-weight baby, and possibly fetal loss.

Hypothyroidism (Underactive Thyroid)

This is much more common than hyperthyroid disease. Hashimoto's thyroiditis is the most common cause of hypothyroidism. Iodine is needed for thyroid hormone production. A reduction of iodized salt in the diet has led to iodine deficiency in a good number of women.

Symptoms of an underactive thyroid include:

- o Fatigue
- o Weight gain
- o Hair loss
- o Dry skin
- o Constipation

If left untreated, there is a higher incidence of preeclampsia, placental abruption, preterm delivery, and a low-birth-weight baby. Hypothyroidism is treated the same way for pregnant women as for non-pregnant women. The use of Levothyroxine is used to normalize TSH levels. This medication is considered safe for use during pregnancy. If you are being treated for thyroid disease, you can expect to have your TSH levels monitored throughout your pregnancy.

CHAPTER 35

Pregnancy and Cancer

Most women do not associate being diagnosed with or treated for cancer during pregnancy as something that could happen to them. Thankfully, cancer during pregnancy is a rare event, occurring only in about 1 in 1,000 pregnancies. Many women who have received a diagnosis of cancer during pregnancy can be treated and still have a normal pregnancy with no significant risk to the fetus. The most common cancers that affect young pregnant women are breast, cervical, colon, Hodgkin's lymphoma, and thyroid cancer. As more women are having children later in life, the number of pregnant women with cancer is rising.

Diagnosing cancer during pregnancy can be difficult because symptoms like headaches, abdominal pain, and rectal and vaginal bleeding can all be attributed to the pregnancy. In addition, swollen breasts during pregnancy make evaluation for pain or a lump difficult. If a suspicious breast lump is found, further testing with ultrasound or an MRI can be done, along with a needle biopsy if necessary. Cervical cancer is often diagnosed from the Pap smear that should be done at the beginning of the first trimester.

Treatment for cancer during pregnancy should balance the best treatment for the mother while protecting the fetus from any adverse effects of chemotherapy or radiation. The issues that go into organizing a plan for treatment include:

○ How far along you are into the pregnancy

○ The type of cancer

○ The stage and progression of the cancer

Chemotherapy and radiation can be toxic to a fetus during the first trimester. Many women will delay treatment until the end of the first trimester when all the major organ systems of the baby are developed.

Chemotherapy can be used during the second and third trimester without harm to the fetus. Radiation may be used in the second or third trimester, depending on the dose and the area of the body being treated. Depending on the stage and progression of the cancer, delivery may take place 4–6 weeks earlier than the due date in order to start a more intensive therapy regimen for the mother. If this is the case, an amniocentesis will be performed to evaluate fetal lung maturity.

The chance of recovery from cancer for a pregnant woman with an early diagnosis is very much the same as for a woman with the same type of cancer who is not pregnant. However, if the diagnosis of cancer is delayed during pregnancy, the overall prognosis would be worse.

In general, pregnancy after cancer is considered safe, and pregnancy does not appear to increase the chance of recurrence. Since recurrences do happen, it is advised that women should wait to have another child for a number of years after receiving treatment, until the risk of recurrence has lessened. Chemotherapy and radiation can be associated with temporary infertility, but more commonly permanent infertility. Before treatment is started, you should discuss this possibility with your doctor.

CHAPTER 36

Cervical Incompetence and Uterine Abnormalities in Pregnancy

One of the top 10 causes of preterm birth and early miscarriage is to be found in abnormalities of the uterus or cervix. The uterus, or womb, is the organ where a woman carries the pregnancy. The baby comes out of the uterus through the cervix into the vagina and out into the world. We all hope that the baby can remain in the uterus and grow until the pregnancy gets beyond 37 weeks, after which time the gestation is considered "full term." Getting to 40 weeks is even better.

 ## Uterine Abnormalities

Nearly 3–4 percent of all reproductive-age women were born with a deformed uterus or uterine abnormality that can result in the birth of a baby before it has completed its full term. About 15–25 percent of women with multiple pregnancy losses can attribute these losses to uterine abnormalities.

Bicornuate uterus

This is the most common abnormality; the uterus is shaped like a heart, with a deep indentation at the top. The baby does not have as much area to grow in as it does in a normally shaped uterus.

Double uterus

This is when the uterus has two cavities. Each cavity may have its own cervix as well. Often, women with a double uterus will get pregnant only on one side. If either uterus is deformed, the risk of preterm birth or miscarriage is increased. Having a double uterus is a very rare abnormality.

Septate uterus

This is when the uterus is divided down the center by a septum, which can extend all the way to the cervix. A septum can be cut out surgically, but there are risks concerning this procedure that should be talked over with your doctor.

Fibroids

Nearly 60 percent of women have fibroids (benign muscle tumors) in the uterus by the age of 35. Fibroids can be a cause of pelvic pain, increased bleeding during your period, and pregnancy complications. Your doctor can determine if you have fibroids either by a pelvic exam or by ultrasound.

Depending on the size and location of these fibroids, a woman may experience the following problems during pregnancy:

- There may be an increased risk of early miscarriage.
- There may be an increased risk of preterm birth.
- There may be episodes of bleeding during the pregnancy.
- There may be increased pain from the fibroid being stretched by the uterine muscle. If pain is severe, your physician may suggest you try a prescription medication called Indocin. This drug is an anti-inflammatory that works very well for this type of pain and is safe for use in pregnancy up to 32 weeks' gestation.
- There may be fibroid growth.
- There may be a higher risk for C-section if the fibroid(s)

blocks the fetal head from moving out of the uterus and into the birth canal.

o   There may be excessive bleeding during and after the birthing process.

Your physician may suggest a dye study, which makes it easier to see what the uterus looks like through an x-ray enhanced with dye. A laparoscope can also be used to look on the inside and outside of your uterus. If you have large or multiple fibroids, your doctor may suggest that they be removed. This can be accomplished with injections, laser, or surgery. Your gynecologist will discuss these options with you. Certainly, if you have a history of miscarriages or early deliveries that your doctor connects to a uterine abnormality, you would benefit from corrective surgery.

Cervical Incompetence

An incompetent cervix is a complication of pregnancy where the muscle that forms the cervix cannot remain closed throughout the pregnancy and begins to shorten and dilate. This inability of the muscle in the cervix to remain closed can result in a premature delivery or a first- or second-trimester pregnancy loss.

The most common causes of incompetent cervix include:
o   Multiple D&Cs
o   Multiple D&Es
o   A LEEP procedure
o   Cervical conization
o   Rapid preterm birth
o   Multiple gestations (twins or more)

If you are at a higher risk of experiencing cervical incompetence, your doctor may wish to follow your cervix with ultrasound, waiting to see whether your cervix shortens. At that point, your doctor may consider putting in a cerclage. The problem encountered when following the length of the cervix by ultrasound is that the cervix can shorten rapidly in one to two days with no warning. If your cervix is going to prematurely dilate, this will likely happen at 18–24 weeks' gestation. Placing a cerclage at this point carries a much greater risk to the pregnancy. There is a higher likelihood of premature rupture of membranes, preterm birth, and pregnancy loss. It is recommended that a cerclage be performed at 11–12 weeks of gestation, before your cervix has a chance to thin out or dilate.

The cerclage procedure is done either under local anesthesia or with a spinal anesthetic in a same-day surgical center. It takes about 10–15 minutes to perform. There are many different ways to place a stitch in the cervix. I personally use the McDonald cervical cerclage, which places a suture around the cervix much like the string in a pouch. There may be some shooting pains in the vagina after the procedure. This usually subsides in one to two weeks. Sex is generally not recommended during this time due to the risk of infection. The stitch is removed at 36 weeks in your doctors office.

The risk of complications is less than 1 percent to the pregnancy, and if it prevents an early delivery, then it was well worth it!

CHAPTER 37

Gastrointestinal and Urinary Problems

Hormone changes in pregnancy can promote gastrointestinal and urinary tract problems that can lead to a host of problems that can plague women at some point during their pregnancy. Below is a list of common problems that a pregnant woman may experience.

Constipation

Constipation in pregnancy affects over half of all women. This can cause pain and discomfort, difficult bowel movements, and hard stools. Excessive straining can also lead to the formation of hemorrhoids.

Constipation in pregnant women is thought to occur due to hormones that relax the intestinal muscle and also from the pressure of the growing uterus on the intestines. Any additional iron supplement you may be taking can also contribute to constipation.

Drinking plenty of water along with a high-fiber diet can help reduce constipation. If you are not getting enough fiber from foods, you can take fiber supplements, such as Metamucil or Citrucel, that are safe to take throughout pregnancy. Exercise can also be very beneficial for the relief of constipation.

Gas and Bloating

Expectant moms often experience an increased amount of intestinal gas and abdominal bloating. This can make you feel uncomfortable and can at times be quite painful.

The increased levels of progesterone during pregnancy can cause the muscles of the body to relax, causing the food that you eat to move slower through your digestive tract. If food leaves your stomach without being fully digested, this will cause gas to accumulate. Eating foods that don't produce excess gas is the best remedy for this problem. You should try to avoid beans, certain vegetables, fried foods, carbonated beverages, and coffee. Eating smaller meals can also be helpful. If dietary changes do not seem to be helping, an anti-gas medication can be used in the second and third trimester. Be sure to check with your healthcare provider before taking any medication.

 ## Heartburn

Heartburn is caused from a backward flow (reflux) of stomach acid moving into the esophagus. Pregnancy causes the stomach muscles to become more relaxed, allowing the stomach acid to reflux more readily, causing moderate to severe pain at any time of the day. Contributing to this tendency, the stomach takes longer to empty during pregnancy, extending the chance for indigestion.

Steps for decreasing indigestion:

- Try very hard to get your weight down prior to the pregnancy. Then do the best you can to keep your weight down by avoiding fats, fast food, and high-sugar-content foods.
- Eat smaller, more frequent meals during the day.
- Drink at least eight cups of water daily.
- Do not smoke (bad for the baby; plus, it increases stomach acid).

- Sit up when you are eating.
- Wait for one hour after eating before you lie down.
- Try not to lie flat on your back.
- Stay away from caffeinated beverages.

Over-the-counter medications like Tums or Mylanta are safe for use during pregnancy.

Hemorrhoids and Pregnancy

As Forest Gump would say, "They go together like peas and carrots!" They are just a big pain in the butt that comes to visit over half of all pregnant women. A woman's blood volume nearly doubles during pregnancy, causing veins in the legs and the vagina and rectum to swell. This can be very painful and result in varicosities (swollen blood vessels) that can contribute to the development or worsening of hemorrhoids. In addition, pressure from the fetus and an enlarged uterus can worsen the pressure to the rectal area.

The following factors increase the risk of getting hemorrhoids:

- Obesity
- Previous history of hemorrhoids
- Constipation
- Low-fiber diet
- Prolonged sitting or standing
- A history of hemorrhoids in past pregnancies

Treatment includes taking stool softeners and laxatives, if needed. Eat food high in fiber or take fiber capsules with your vitamin each day. Take sitz baths in warm water one to two times a day. If the hemorrhoids are severe and these treatments are not helping, then have your obstetrician refer you to a colorectal surgeon for evaluation and treatment. These treatments are safe during the pregnancy and have no effect on the unborn child.

Urinary Tract Infection (UTI)

Women often have problems throughout their pregnancy with their bladder and urinary tract because being pregnant slows down the movement of urine from the kidneys to the bladder. This can cause minor to serious infections and can increase uterine contractions and pelvic pain. Urine can pool in the bladder, often remaining there even after you empty it. This increases the risk of bacteria multiplying to infection status, causing pelvic pain and burning when you urinate. Over 5 percent of all pregnant women get at least one UTI during their pregnancy.

Making the diagnosis is easy with a sample of urine in your doctor's office. Treatment with an antibiotic is usually the only treatment needed, unless some pain relief is also necessary. Antibiotics for a UTI are safe to take during pregnancy.

Steps to prevent urinary infections:

o Drink plenty of fluids, especially water. This helps wash out the kidneys and bladder, and it reduces the chance of bacteria making your bladder their home.

o Avoid coffee and tea, which can increase irritation in the bladder.

o Completely empty your bladder every time you urinate. If you feel you still have some urine left after five or 10 minutes, then go a second time.

o Keep your vaginal and rectal areas very clean.

o Maintain a very healthy diet, as we have discussed throughout this book.

If you think that you have a UTI, but you also have a fever, then you may have an infection in your kidneys. This is a different infection and can be dangerous and lead to preterm labor and early delivery. Contact your doctor for a complete evaluation as soon as possible.

Urinary Incontinence

During pregnancy, many women experience pressure on the bladder from the growing uterus and urine leaks due to a general relaxing of the muscles in the pelvic region. Leaking will often happen after sneezing, coughing, laughing, and lifting something heavy. Emptying your bladder frequently and performing kegel exercises (see chapter 72) may keep you from having these "little accidents." If you find yourself leaking urine more often than you would like, you might consider wearing a panty liner during the day.

CHAPTER 38

Seizure Disorders

Epilepsy and other neurological disorders can cause seizures. The majority of people with adult seizures take daily medication to control them. Any woman with a seizure disorder should see her neurologist prior to getting pregnant. You will want your condition to be under the best control possible, preferably on a single-use agent. During pregnancy, blood levels of medications can change, so it is important to make certain you are on the correct dose throughout your pregnancy. It is very important not to stop taking your anticonvulsant medication, as having a seizure can cause harm to the baby.

Pregnancy can be associated with both an increase and a decrease in seizure activity. Nearly one-third of women with epilepsy in pregnancy have an increase in seizure activity, while the other two-thirds either have no change or a decrease. Those women who are in poor control of their seizures normally will also have difficulty controlling them during their pregnancy.

If you have a seizure disorder, the risk of congenital fetal abnormalities is about 2 percent, *which is double the risk in the general population*. If you are taking medication for seizure disorders, the risk of having a baby with a birth defect increases to about 4 percent. The most common birth defects seen from anti-epileptic drugs are neural tube defects, cleft lip/palate, and congenital heart disease. It is recommended that the fetus have a detailed ultrasound and fetal echocardiogram evaluation by a high-risk obstetrician. The majority of women who are treated for seizures will have normal pregnancies and healthy babies.

Seizures are increased in women with the following problems:

- A family history of seizure disorders
- Excess alcohol abuse
- Drug abuse
- Low blood sugar
- Prior head injury

CHAPTER 39

Asthma

Asthma is a chronic lung disease that inflames and narrows the airways. Asthma symptoms, including coughing, wheezing, and chest tightness, are common during an asthma attack.

If you have suffered with asthma in the past, you should make an appointment with the provider who has treated you for your condition as soon as you find out you are pregnant. This way, you can be sure you have any medications you may need. Make sure that your ob/gyn provider is also aware that you are being treated or have been treated in the past for asthma.

During pregnancy, your immune system can be suppressed and allergies and upper respiratory viral infections seen more frequently. It is important to remember that your unborn baby relies on the air you breathe to supply its oxygen. When you have an asthma attack, the baby might not get enough oxygen, which can be very dangerous for its development.

Many women find that their asthma and allergies get much better during pregnancy. If you are one of these women, that is great. If you are not one of these women, do not fret. Many asthma medications are safe to take during pregnancy.

Women with uncontrolled asthma are also much more likely to have pregnancy complications, such as high blood pressure and premature delivery. If you have an asthma attack and find your medication is not doing the job, make sure to contact your doctor as soon as possible.

 ## Reminders to Minimize Asthma Attacks:

- Try to stay away from any triggers that may have caused your attacks in the past.

- Stay away from areas where chemicals are being used. If you are painting the baby's room, make sure there is adequate ventilation.

- If your attacks have ever been exercise-induced, do only light exercises that don't get you out of breath.

- As long as your asthma stays well under control during your pregnancy, you should not experience any problems.

CHAPTER 40

Multiple Sclerosis

Multiple Sclerosis (MS) is an autoimmune disorder that can frequently affect women during their reproductive years. Many years ago, women were discouraged from having children if they had multiple sclerosis. That is no longer the case. Studies now show that pregnancy is actually protective for women with MS.

Here are some common questions patients with MS ask regarding their pregnancy:

Are pregnancy complications more likely if you have MS?

Women can usually progress normally through pregnancy and have a normal full-term birth. There is no evidence that MS is linked to any specific problems with pregnancy.

Will MS symptoms get worse during pregnancy?

Women with MS often say they feel better. Furthermore, they often have few symptoms of the disease while they are pregnant. Pregnancy seems to have a protective effect, possibly because pregnancy reduces immune activity, and levels of natural steroids are higher. MS relapses are greatly reduced during pregnancy, especially in the second and third trimester.

❓ What about treatment for MS during pregnancy?

If you are currently on any type of treatment, you will probably be advised to stop taking it while trying to conceive as well as throughout the pregnancy. Your neurologist will likely be involved in your pregnancy regarding treatment options, monitoring your MS while you are pregnant. Your primary ob/gyn may also have you consult a high-risk OB specialist to see you during your pregnancy.

❓ Can you use spinal anesthesia during delivery?

Some neurologists advise against using an epidural because they believe there is a greater risk of complication. However, studies show women with MS who had epidurals did not have a higher rate of relapse than those who did not. The form of anesthesia to be used should be discussed with both your obstetrician and your neurologist toward the end of your pregnancy.

❓ Will I have a relapse after delivery?

Your risk of relapse in the first six months after delivery is somewhere between 20 and 40 percent. Studies have shown that a dose of intravenous immunoglobulin (IVIG) given to women immediately following delivery greatly reduces the chance of a relapse.

❓ Will my child develop MS?

MS is not directly inherited. Evidence does show that a child born to a parent with MS has a 20 percent chance of someday developing MS themselves.

CHAPTER 41

Lupus

Lupus is an autoimmune disease that primarily affects women between their 20s and 40s. Many years ago, it was thought that women who had lupus could not or should not become pregnant. If you have lupus and are thinking of becoming pregnant, it is best to schedule a pre-pregnancy consultation with your healthcare provider. Today, with the use of advanced fetal testing and evaluation of the mother, about 50 percent of women with lupus can have a completely normal pregnancy.

The best outcomes are achieved in women who conceive after having their symptoms in remission for at least six months. Getting pregnant when your disease is active can result in miscarriage, stillbirth, or pregnancy complications. Babies born to mothers with lupus are *not* at an increased risk of birth defects.

Flare-ups that do develop often occur in the first or second trimester and are usually mild. Use of steroids may be necessary if symptoms become worse during the pregnancy. Prednisone is usually prescribed and is safe to take during pregnancy.

It is very important that your pregnancy be monitored by a high-risk specialist. Pregnant women with lupus are more likely to suffer from hypertension, fetal growth restriction, and preterm delivery. Close evaluations with antenatal testing should occur weekly in the last six weeks of pregnancy.

Approximately one-third of babies born to women with lupus will contract neonatal lupus. This condition is not particularly serious and is usually accompanied by a rash that clears up on its own. *Of these babies, 1 percent may develop neonatal heart block, which is a slowing of the newborn's heart rate and may require a pacemaker for a short period of time.*

CHAPTER 42

Depression and Anxiety Disorder in Pregnancy

Psychiatric disorders, such as depression and anxiety disorder, affect more than 500,000 pregnant women yearly. Many of these women have already been diagnosed and/or treated prior to getting pregnant. Other women will experience symptoms for the very first time during a pregnancy. About one-third of these women will be on some type of medication during their pregnancy to treat symptoms.

 ## Signs of depression and anxiety disorder include:

- Severe unhappiness
- Fatigue
- Insomnia
- Poor appetite
- Heart palpitations
- Fear of losing control
- Mood swings

Pregnancy can be a time filled with much stress and anxiety. Coupled with changing hormones experienced during pregnancy, it can make a woman more prone to changes in mood and feelings of sadness. These types of feelings can often be a crushing blow to women who have never felt them before.

Many women will choose to suffer in silence, feeling guilty because this is supposed to be a happy time in their life. However, you should not feel alone, as many women suffer through the same exact feelings you are experiencing.

The good news is there is help to treat these symptoms. There are a number of medications that are safe to take during pregnancy. Selective serotonin re-uptake inhibitors (SSRIs) are frequently used and are relatively safe to take throughout pregnancy. The risks of not taking these medications—if they relieve symptoms of depression and anxiety—are far greater than the risks associated with stopping the medications, which include preterm delivery and other pregnancy-related complications.

If left untreated, depression and other mood disorders can cause serious medical and pregnancy-related problems for both the mom and the unborn baby. Poor eating habits, irregular sleep, anxiety, and high levels of stress lead to these serious problems. Postpartum depression is also more likely to occur if symptoms are not treated before delivery.

If you have ever been treated for anxiety, depression, or other psychological illnesses and are planning on getting pregnant, see the doctor who treated you in the past and make a plan for how you will be treated during and after your pregnancy. Let your ob/gyn caregiver know what medications you are on, or have been on in the past, and how they may have helped you.

COMPLICATIONS OF PREGNANCY

CHAPTER 43

High Blood Pressure and Preeclampsia

Chronic high blood pressure prior to pregnancy is often associated with a family history of high blood pressure, being overweight, being over age 35, and smoking cigarettes. It is important to have your blood pressure under control. Talk to your family doctor or obstetrician to be sure you are on medications that are safe in pregnancy. Chronic high blood pressure is common in pregnant women. About 1 in 20 pregnant women have chronic hypertension prior to getting pregnant.

Women who start out with normal blood pressure values and then have high blood pressure values between 20 weeks and term are called pregnancy-induced hypertensives. These women may go on to develop preeclampsia.

Following are common questions regarding your blood pressure and your pregnancy:

❓ Can high blood pressure cause problems during the pregnancy for my baby and me?

○ Chronic high blood pressure can increase the risk of premature birth, growth restriction of the fetus (small baby), stillbirth (fetal demise), placental problems (abruption or premature aging), and having a C-section.

○ With really high blood pressure that is not well

controlled, nearly one in three women have a small baby, and two in three women have an early delivery.

o Women with chronic high blood pressure have a 20–50 percent risk of getting preeclampsia, which results in higher risks for problems in the second and third trimesters to both the mother and the baby.

What is preeclampsia?

Preeclampsia is unique to pregnancy and is a combination of high blood pressure, changes in blood chemistry values, and protein in the urine after the second trimester. It can cause seizures in the mother and may require an immediate delivery.

Who usually gets preeclampsia?

o Seven out of every 100 pregnant women get preeclampsia.

o It happens more often in the first pregnancy.

o Preeclampsia happens more often in multiple gestations.

o Women who have diabetes are more likely to get preeclampsia.

o Teenagers and women over 30 are at higher risk of getting preeclampsia.

o Women with a history of hypertension or kidney disease are at higher risk.

If I have preeclampsia, do I need to be delivered?

Yes. Delivery is often necessary within days to a week or two depending on how far you are into your third trimester. Both you and your baby can be in serious danger if you are not delivered soon after preeclampsia is diagnosed. Hospitalization may be necessary before delivery if you are less than 34 weeks, to give the baby the benefit of steroids for faster lung development.

⍰ How do hypertension and preeclampsia hurt my baby in the womb?

High blood pressure can reduce blood flow, which will reduce oxygen to the placenta. The baby needs oxygen for growth and good health in the womb.

⍰ What can be done to watch my baby in case problems occur?

- Ultrasound evaluation, which looks at the baby's growth and movement, can be done frequently. This is called growth assessment and antenatal testing.
- In addition, a study called a "Doppler" can make sure the baby is getting enough oxygen from the placenta.

Check with your obstetrician about these tests, which are usually started at about 32 weeks of gestation.

⍰ What problems could occur if my blood pressure remains out of control?

- A continued rising blood pressure and a possible early delivery
- Headaches
- Swelling in the face and hands
- Blurred vision
- Pain in the upper right abdominal area below your ribs
- Cramps and vaginal bleeding
- Risk of preeclampsia

❔ What do ob/gyn doctors suggest for women who have chronic high blood pressure and are planning a pregnancy?

o   Have a pre-pregnancy consultation with your OB doctor or a high-risk specialist before becoming pregnant.

o   The drugs Methyldopa and Labetalol are the two most common drugs used for women with high blood pressure planning a pregnancy. These drugs are safe to use in pregnancy.

❔ What else can I do to help my blood pressure?

o   Drink plenty of water.

o   Use no added salt, and stay away from food with a high salt content.

o   Stay away from "fast food."

o   Get plenty of rest (six to eight hours of sleep per night).

o   Try to lower daily stress.

o   Maintain a sensible, healthy diet and a moderate plan for exercise—even 20 minutes walking four days per week will help lower your blood pressure.

Chronic high blood pressure and preeclampsia both involve your blood pressure being high but are often handled differently. You should be checked carefully at each prenatal visit for blood pressure values. Blood pressure that remains high beyond six weeks after birth may mean that you have chronic hypertension and need long-term treatment.

Other Blood Pressure Issues

Low Blood Pressure

Low blood pressure occurs much less frequently than high blood pressure during pregnancy and does not generally cause any serious complications to the pregnancy. Having low blood pressure will more likely cause a mom-to-be to feel dizzy, lightheaded, and short of breath. The most common causes for low blood pressure during pregnancy are dehydration and extra pressure on large blood vessels like the aorta and vena cava, caused by the growing fetus. The best ways to avoid having low blood pressure—especially during the second and third trimesters—are to drink at least eight cups of water daily, and lay on your side, rather than flat on your back. Keeping your blood pressure at a normal level will ensure that the baby is getting an adequate amount of oxygen and nutrients.

CHAPTER 44

Diabetes

One of the most serious medical epidemics in the United States is the dramatic increase in type 2 diabetes. This is mainly due to very poor eating habits coupled with the epidemic of obesity and limited physical activity. The age of onset has decreased to the 30s and 40s for both men and women. There are tens of thousands of people who are type 2 diabetics and have not yet been diagnosed.

If you have type 1 or 2 diabetes and are on medication, you should have already seen a specialist prior to getting pregnant. If that did not happen, then you may need a high-risk specialist as a consultant or as your primary delivering obstetrician. Your medications, oral or injected insulin, should be managed on a weekly basis.

Women who have risk factors like diabetes in the family, advanced maternal age (over 35), obesity (over 20 percent above ideal body weight), and prior pregnancy with gestational diabetes should have counseling and careful evaluation prior to their next pregnancy. In addition, improved dietary habits and an exercise program should be started as well.

A pregnant woman with diabetes who is in good control of her blood sugar values with a proper diet can usually have as uneventful and normal a pregnancy as a woman without diabetes. However, if a woman gets pregnant while in poor control of her blood sugar, the fetus is at high risk for birth defects (especially heart defects), preterm birth, preeclampsia, and stillbirth.

Pregnancy often makes diabetes difficult to control because the pregnancy hormones reduce the effectiveness of the body's insulin. The pancreas has to try to keep up with the increased requirements for insulin as the pregnancy progresses. Often, with increased body weight and/or a family history of diabetes coupled with age, the risk of becoming diabetic during the pregnancy increases.

 ## Three Types of Diabetes

1. **Gestational diabetes** is diabetes that occurs during the second half of the pregnancy and is usually diagnosed after week 28 by a glucose tolerance test.

2. **Type 1 or juvenile diabetes** occurs at a very young age and is caused by an autoimmune condition that results in the destruction of the pancreas cells that produce insulin, leading to a dependence on daily insulin.

3. **Type 2 adult-onset diabetes** is more common today in younger adults and is more common today in pregnancy than it was years ago.

 ## What You Should Know about Gestational Diabetes

○ You may be asked to see a high-risk obstetrician for special counseling and care. Your doctor will discuss this with you.

○ The most common diabetes in pregnancy (90 percent) is gestational diabetes, which affects 50,000–100,000 pregnant women yearly in the United States.

○ Over 50 percent of women with gestational diabetes

eventually get type 2 diabetes, usually within 10–15 years.

o   Many of the women today who are diagnosed as "gestational diabetics" during their pregnancy had diabetes before the pregnancy started. This is really type 2 adult diabetes.

o   One major risk to poorly controlled gestational diabetes is having a large baby. This can increase the risk of injury to the baby during the birthing process. These babies are also at risk for respiratory and cardiac problems and often spend time in the high-risk nursery.

o   Gestational diabetes usually does not have any signs or symptoms. This is why a screening test (glucose tolerance test) is done between week 26 and week 28 by your doctor.

o   If you were just diagnosed as a gestational diabetic, you need to follow a special diet that is a healthy, balanced diet, and low in sugar and fats.

o   Women with gestational diabetes should be tested three to six months after delivery with a two-hour glucose tolerance test.

 ## Risks Associated with Diabetes during Pregnancy

Diabetes in pregnancy contributes to and may cause the following:

o   Eye damage (retina), short term and long term (mother)

o   Increased risk of kidney damage (mother)

o   Increased risk of preterm delivery

o   Chronic hypertension (mother)

o   Preeclampsia

- Increased risk of birth defects (especially congenital heart disease)
- Increase in stillbirths
- Increased risk of C-section
- Higher-birth-weight baby
- Shoulder dystocia

 ## Controlling Diabetes during Pregnancy

The basics for control of diabetes in pregnancy include the following:

Blood Sugar Monitoring

Discuss with your doctor how often you need blood sugar testing. If you are on insulin, you need a fasting blood sugar in the morning. Then you should record a blood sugar value two hours after each meal, totaling four blood sugar values per day.

Dietary Plan

You need to have a carefully planned diet so that you have a wide variety of foods to choose from that will keep your blood sugar in good control. Your total calories per day will depend on your weight and your blood sugar values.

Exercise

It is important to get some exercise three to four days per week. I favor walking. Always make sure to keep water and a healthy snack with you. If you feel you need a healthy snack before you take a walk, go right ahead.

Medication

If diet and exercise are not adequately controlling your blood sugar, you may be placed on oral medication or insulin.

Gaining or Losing Weight during Pregnancy

Most women should gain weight during their pregnancy, but if you are on a diet for diabetes, you may not gain much weight. In fact, you can even lose weight during certain weeks. Women who are seriously overweight can go through the pregnancy gaining only 10–15 pounds, and the fetus will be at no risk. Women on a diabetic diet will often slow down in weight gain during the third trimester. This also carries no risk to the fetus.

Fetal Antenatal Testing

All women with diabetes, no matter which type, must have weekly or twice-weekly fetal testing with a high-risk specialist for fetal well-being. These tests can include a non-stress test, which is a 20-minute monitor strip that measures the baby's heartbeat. A biophysical profile can include the non-stress test. This test also measures the amniotic fluid around the baby, the baby's movements, and fetal breathing. In addition, measuring blood flow through the umbilical cord can detect normal or abnormal oxygen transport to the baby from the placenta.

Planning Delivery

How good your blood sugar control has been, as well as what type of diabetes you have, will determine what week of gestation delivery should occur. Most women with type 1 or 2 diabetes are delivered by 38–39 weeks. Women with well-controlled gestational diabetes can often go to 41 weeks' gestation before delivery. If the baby is large (ultrasound-estimated weight), your doctor will talk with you about a scheduled C-section.

The Future of Diagnosing and Treating Diabetes in Pregnancy

Future Testing

Because adult-onset diabetes is becoming an epidemic in the young adult population, obstetricians will soon be testing women at risk early in the first trimester. Currently, all women are tested in the 28th week of pregnancy with a glucose tolerance test. If testing reveals high blood sugar levels, a woman is often labeled as a gestational diabetic. However, some of these women were already diabetic before the pregnancy.

A blood test called hemoglobin A1C can be used to check if a person's blood sugar has been elevated for the past three months. Using hemoglobin A1C testing early in pregnancy will make certain a woman does not have diabetes prior to pregnancy.

In addition, this testing will make sure that the patient understands that she is affected with a condition that will require further treatment and doesn't just have a condition that goes away after pregnancy.

Future Treatment

Diabetes that is not controlled well during pregnancy can be very dangerous. Many women, especially women with insulin-dependent diabetes, have frequently been noncompliant with keeping their blood sugar controlled because of not wanting to use needles and syringes.

A new system has been developed that will allow a pregnant women to easily administer insulin to herself in a painless way. The OmniPod insulin management system permits you to have the advantage of an insulin pump without the tubing and cumbersome size of a traditional insulin pump. A small pod (the size of half an egg) with a catheter and micro-needle is placed on a specific location on the skin, and then the needle is removed. This pod stays in place for three days and dispenses insulin 24 hours a day with extra insulin at mealtime. After three days, it is removed and replaced with a new pod. This device keeps blood sugar levels controlled and is very easy to use. Women using such a device have a lower hemoglobin A1C and fewer complications during pregnancy.

CHAPTER 45

Amniotic Fluid: Too Little (Oligohydramnios) or Too Much (Polyhydramnios)

Amniotic fluid is an important part of pregnancy and fetal development. This fluid helps protect your baby while still inside and also plays an important role in the development of certain internal organs. Amniotic fluid problems occur in about 5–10 percent of pregnancies.

 ## Oligohydramnios (insufficiency)

Olighydramnios is when there is a less than normal amount of amniotic fluid surrounding the baby. This is usually seen in the second and third trimesters. In the second trimester, low amniotic fluid can result from fetal kidney disease, major birth defects, or chronic hypertension in the mother. The condition can also be seen with antiphospholipid syndrome.

After 16 weeks' gestation, amniotic fluid is composed of fetal urine. If the fetus has a serious kidney defect, less urine might be produced. This can be detected by ultrasound. The fetus urinates throughout the second and third trimester and then swallows the urine, which is critical to fetal lung development.

A decrease in amniotic fluid *in the third trimester* is more likely to be caused by chronic hypertension, fetal growth restriction, antiphospholipid syndrome, and preterm rupture of the membranes. *If you think you may have ruptured your water bag, call your doctor immediately.*

Is it true that when the amniotic fluid is low around the baby, my doctor may decide to replace the fluid so that my pregnancy can continue safely until my due date?

No, that is not true. Replacing the amniotic fluid does not reduce the risk of low fluid and is not a treatment for oligohydramnios. Depending on other risk factors, your doctor may decide to deliver the baby, hospitalize you for monitoring, or place you on bed rest with frequent ultrasound evaluations of the amount of amniotic fluid. If the low fluid is a result of ruptured membranes, your doctor will most likely deliver you within a short time.

 ## Polyhydramnios (overabundance)

Polyhydramnios is when there is an excess amount of amniotic fluid, often resulting from a large baby, poorly controlled diabetes, or—rarely—a blockage in the throat of the fetus restricting normal swallowing of the fluid. Over 98 percent of excessive amniotic fluid results from excess urine production, which can come from a large baby or as a result of high fetal blood sugar related to the mother's diabetes.

Polyhydramnios can result in a higher risk for a C-section and excessive postpartum bleeding due to the extra fluid over-distending the uterus. If the extra fluid is from high blood sugar, the newborn baby may be placed in the neonatal intensive care unit (NICU) for one to two days to control low blood sugar changes that could cause seizures.

Polyhydramnios can also put you at higher risk for premature labor and delivery, premature rupture of the membranes, and placental separation or abruption.

Excessive amniotic fluid can cause these symptoms:

- Shortness of breath
- Getting very big in a short period of time
- Indigestion
- Contractions

Can my doctor remove this extra fluid so that I will feel better?

The only time we would remove amniotic fluid from around the baby in this situation is if the amount of fluid was so great that the risk of early delivery was high. This happens only in about 1 percent of all cases of polyhydramnios. Removed fluid would re-accumulate in just a few days. Most of the time, extra fluid is just monitored by your doctor, and it usually decreases naturally toward the end of the pregnancy.

CHAPTER 46

Intrauterine Growth Restriction

Intrauterine growth restriction is a term that refers to babies who slow down in growth and are smaller in size than the average baby in the second and third trimesters. In the United States, there are about 50,000 babies born at term per year with a birth weight of less than five and a half pounds (10th percentile).

 Causes of growth restriction include:

- ○ High blood pressure (hypertension)
- ○ Cigarette smoking
- ○ Type 1 diabetes (juvenile)
- ○ Poor weight gain/low maternal body weight
- ○ Alcohol or drug abuse
- ○ Placental abnormalities
- ○ Birth defects
- ○ Multiple gestation
- ○ Antiphospholipid antibody syndrome
- ○ Infections like rubella, CMV, or toxoplasmosis
- ○ Advanced maternal age (over 35)

- o   Poor nutrition
- o   Prior small baby at term

In women carrying twins, there usually is a difference in the size between the two babies. Couples usually think that the smaller baby may need extra pediatric care. However, if the twins are born prematurely, the smaller baby is usually more mature than the large twin because babies that are smaller in the womb have more rapid lung maturity than babies of normal weight.

A pregnancy where intrauterine growth restriction is suspected will be followed closely by your doctor with ultrasound growth assessment and fetal well-being tests. In addition, if a reason for the smaller baby is suspected, certain treatments may be added. This can include blood pressure medication, aspirin, heparin, or giving up smoking. Sometimes, improved nutrition can help to improve fetal growth.

Nonetheless, it is good to avoid fetal growth restrictions, and the best way to do that is to stop smoking, maintain normal blood pressure, and have a healthy diet.

CHAPTER 47

Multiple Gestations

The incidence of multiple births has been on the rise for the past 10–20 years, especially due to the use of assisted reproductive technology. In addition, the number of multiple births has increased because many more women over the age of 35 are having children. Women over 35 are more likely to expel more than one egg that can be fertilized during an ovulation cycle.

What You Should Know about Multiple Gestations:

o   Women carrying multiples carry a significant risk for developing high blood pressure, diabetes, preterm labor, premature delivery, fetal growth problems, preeclampsia, and more severe nausea and vomiting.

o   Multiple gestations have a naturally higher risk of birth defects. Your risk *doubles* with twins, *triples* with triplets, and so on. Close evaluation by a high-risk obstetrician is strongly suggested. Prenatal diagnosis (CVS or amniocentesis) should be discussed during the early part of the pregnancy.

o   An ultrasound exam can usually determine if the twins are identical or fraternal.

- Your office visits will be more frequent when carrying multiples.

- Expectant moms with twins or more are usually put on a higher-calorie diet throughout the pregnancy.

- Women of advanced maternal age (over 35) have a higher complication rate when carrying multiples.

- Anemia is more common in multiples, so it is recommended that you take 60–100 milligrams of additional iron.

- Multiples conceived by using either super-ovulation drugs or in vitro fertilization (IVF) are in much greater danger of having medical and obstetrical complications and should be seen by a high-risk specialist during the pregnancy.

- About 20 percent of twins are born prematurely (before 37 weeks), and over 95 percent of triplets are born early.

- Close observation by ultrasound for fetal growth of the twins or triplets is recommended.

- Fewer than 50 percent of twins are delivered vaginally, due to presentation of the babies or other obstetrical and medical complications.

I've heard of twin-twin transfusion syndrome. Am I at risk for this complication, and what can be done if my babies have it?

Twin-twin transfusion syndrome (TTTS) is when a set of identical twins' blood supply is connected. One baby will receive more blood than the other baby, resulting in anemia in the smaller baby and excessive blood volume in the larger baby. Twin-twin transfusion syndrome occurs only in 10 percent of identical twins. As a high-risk obstetrician, I see only one to two cases of TTTS per year, while I see over 40 multiples or more yearly. Most couples with multiples do not have to worry about this complication occurring in identical twins because the vast majority of twins

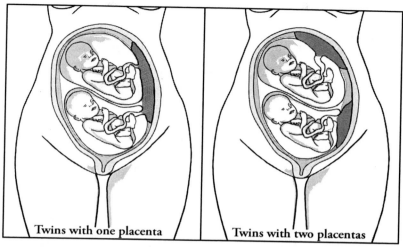

Twins with one placenta | Twins with two placentas

are fraternal and each has its own placenta. Twins that share a single placenta are at a small risk (10 percent) of one of the babies getting more blood than the other, causing that baby to be larger than the other.

High-risk fetal surgical centers are now treating this complication with ultrasound-guided laser treatment. The blood vessels in the placenta that are causing the misdirection of blood are fixed so that each baby can resume normal growth while still sharing the same placenta. There are only a few centers in the United States that provide this unique and highly technical procedure.

If you are told that your identical twins may have twin-twin transfusion syndrome (TTTS), see a maternal-fetal medicine specialist to evaluate your pregnancy and refer you to the proper medical center for possible treatment. Pregnancies with TTTS that go untreated can result in very serious complications to both babies. The treatment for TTTS also carries significant risks.

What is a vanishing twin?

A vanishing twin usually happens in the first trimester, where one of the babies is lost and the surviving twin continues to progress normally throughout the pregnancy. The twin that is lost will be absorbed and not be present at birth. Occasionally, a twin pregnancy will lose one of the babies after the first trimester. When this happens, the baby that has died remains in the uterus and will be delivered when the viable baby delivers. This problem poses little risk to the pregnancy.

I do not want to have a C-section and would like to attempt a vaginal birth. Can I insist on this with my doctor?

You need to discuss your feelings about your delivery early on with your doctor. Today, doctors are more cautious with multiples, and many more are pushing for delivery by C-section rather than the vaginal route. If your first baby is head first, a good number of obstetricians will attempt a vaginal birth. However, you will be warned that the second baby may have to be delivered by C-section.

What if one of the babies is bigger than the other? Is that normal?

Certainly it is! The majority of multiple births do not have babies that weigh the same. If their weights become greater than 20 percent apart, your doctor may monitor you more closely.

What's the difference between fraternal and identical twins?

Fraternal twins come from two eggs that get fertilized at the same time by two different sperm. Each baby has its own placenta and blood supply. This is the safest type of twins to have and is by far the most common. You are more likely to have fraternal twins as you get older. In addition, if twins run on your mother's side of the family, you are more likely to have twins.

Identical twins result from one fertilized egg that splits into two during the first few days of gestation, resulting in twins that have identical sets of DNA and usually look the same as well. The safest identical twins are those that split apart three to eight days in and have their own sacs. Identical twins that do not split until 8–13 days in the womb will share the same sac and have a higher risk of getting tangled in each other's umbilical cords. However, this does not occur very often.

Can twins switch position in the womb where baby A becomes baby B and visa versa?

No, that cannot happen because the placenta of each baby implants in a certain area of the uterus and, like the roots of a tree, can never move. Twin A is the one nearer to the cervix and will be there until delivery. With triplets, the highest one is baby C, and then baby A and B are identified like twins with baby A nearest to the cervix.

Should I see a high-risk obstetrician for my entire pregnancy?

No, this is probably not necessary. Often, seeing a high-risk obstetrician as a consultant along with your primary obstetrician is perfectly fine. If problems arise either medically or related to the pregnancy, your obstetrician may transfer you to the care of a high-risk specialist for the remainder of your care and delivery. This is between you and your primary obstetrician.

How much weight should I gain with twins and triplets?

Women who are near normal weight should gain about 40-plus pounds with twins and 45–50 pounds with triplets. Women who are moderately overweight may gain 25–35 pounds with twins and 35–40 pounds with triplets. Morbidly obese women (over

250 pounds) should gain no more than 25 pounds with multiples, or less.

What are the best exercises to do if I am having two or three at once?

The same exercises you would do if you were carrying one! Walking is always great, as are stretching and yoga.

CHAPTER 48

Viruses and Infections

Viruses and infections are the most common reasons for getting a phone call, day or night, from a patient. Colds, upset stomachs with diarrhea, and vomiting are very common and unlikely to cause any danger to you or your baby. However, there are some less common infections that can sometimes pose dangers to the baby. These are discussed below.

 ## Colds and Upper-Respiratory Infections

Most adults get one to two colds per year, and you're likely to have an upper-respiratory infection with a rhinovirus during the course of your pregnancy. You should treat yourself as you would if you were not pregnant. Most over-the-counter decongestants and cold medications are safe and rated class B by the Food and Drug Administration (FDA), which means there is no evidence that the fetus is in any danger with use of these medications. However, always check with your caregiver before taking these or any medications. If you develop a low-grade fever (less than 101°F), treat the temperature with common medications like acetaminophen. Fevers greater than 102°F are of more concern though, and you should contact your doctor.

Gastrointestinal Infections

G.I. viruses are also common during pregnancy, and the best treatment is to stay hydrated and eat a very bland diet of rice, crackers, and soups. Avoid hard-to-digest and spicy foods for a few days. Over-the-counter medications for an upset stomach are fine to take during your pregnancy. Contact your doctor if you are vomiting, having diarrhea, and cannot hold any food or drink without vomiting. You do not want to get dehydrated.

 ## Influenza

Getting the flu during your pregnancy can be dangerous to both you and your baby. If you have a history of asthma, respiratory illnesses, smoke, or are near children or people at risk for the flu, I would recommend that you get the yearly influenza vaccine. The flu shot is safe to take during your pregnancy.

 ## Bladder and Kidney Infections

One in 15–20 women frequently get urinary tract infections (UTI) in pregnancy (see chapter 37). Often, women cannot completely empty their bladder, and that extra urine can get infected. A burning sensation at the end of urinating is a sign of a possible infection, as is very frequent urination. Never take an antibiotic before getting a urine culture that confirms an infection. Wash daily (a shower is preferred) and avoid bubble baths, shower gels, detergents, and chlorinated pools. If an untreated UTI is ignored, the infection can elevate to the kidneys, causing a kidney infection with a fever. Kidney infection can lead to premature labor. If you think you have a bladder problem, or you have a fever and are aching in your lower back, get in touch with your doctor for an evaluation.

Vaginal Infections

Vaginal infections are very common in pregnancy. This is due to your depressed immunity and increased vaginal mucus. Things that contribute to an increase in vaginal infections include douching, taking baths, going into the ocean, having sexual intercourse, and using perfumed sprays. Most vaginal infections will have a foul odor, a gray or whitish appearance, and burn or itch. *Bacterial vaginal infections can be linked to a higher risk of preterm rupture of membranes, amniotic fluid infection, first trimester pregnancy loss, and preterm birth.* Contact your doctor for a visit if you feel you have a vaginal infection. Antibiotics can be given to cure the infection in 7–10 days.

 ## Yeast infections

Yeast infections (candidiasis) are a result of an organism called candida albicans, which is found naturally in the vagina in over one-third of all women. In pregnancy, the increased estrogen levels often throw off the natural (good) bacteria, thus allowing some organisms like yeast to overgrow. Candida may increase in number, causing an infection that can present with a thick, white discharge, itching, burning, and redness in the vagina and on the labia and vulva. This infection can be safely treated during pregnancy with suppositories, vaginal creams, or pills prescribed by your doctor. To help prevent a yeast infection, eat yogurt, use underwear with a cotton crotch, and avoid staying in a wet bathing suit or sweaty workout clothes.

 ## Fifth Disease (parvovirus B19)

This is a very common infection seen in many school-aged children that causes a bright red rash on the cheeks. Most kids with this infection will feel fine. Adults can get this disease also and will present with very sore joints, but usually no rash. Once you have had this infection, you usually won't get it again. Fifth disease is very contagious and not uncommon for pregnant women to contract. In rare cases, the fetus will suffer severe fetal anemia, which can cause the baby to die in the womb. Therefore, if the mother is found to have a first-time case of fifth disease, she should see a high-risk obstetrician for evaluation of the fetus. I have seen many women with a first-time case of parvovirus B19 and have checked several babies for anemia by sampling the fetal blood through the umbilical cord (cordocentesis). On two occasions, I had to transfuse the babies in the womb. Both did well after birth.

 ## Cytomegalovirus (CMV)

CMV is a very common virus in adults. Most adults get exposed as children or young adults. If you are positive for CMV virus, there is no risk to the fetus. Even if you contract CMV virus for the first time during pregnancy, there is a very low risk of causing any problems to the baby. Testing for CMV is not routine, and if you want to know whether or not you have been exposed and are immune, have your doctor test you. If you are negative, the best way to prevent contracting CMV is to wash your hands often, especially if you are frequently around young children.

 ## Chickenpox (varicella)

If you have been exposed to chickenpox and are not immune, contact your doctor for a shot (VZIG) to boost your own body's immunity. Very bad respiratory infections can occur in the mother if chickenpox goes untreated. The problem is only serious for the fetus if and when the mom gets chickenpox one to two weeks before delivery.

 ## Hepatitis

There are four kinds of hepatitis—A, B, C, and D. The most dangerous type is hepatitis B or HBV.

Risk factors for HBV include:

- Use of needles to inject street drugs
- Multiple sex partners
- Living with someone affected with HBV
- Working with a high-risk population

A mother with HBV has a 70–80 percent chance of transmitting the virus to the newborn. Testing a mother for HBV should be done at the beginning of each pregnancy. Symptoms are non-specific and hard to identify, but include nausea and vomiting, which is very common in pregnancy anyway.

All teens and adults should get the vaccination if there is a high risk for HBV. If you think you have been exposed during pregnancy, you can receive the vaccine. If you were exposed during the pregnancy and test positive, you can get a hepatitis B immunization that will make the illness mild and reduce any severe "flu-like" symptoms. If you get the vaccine and treatment, the risk of passing the hepatitis to the fetus is reduced from 80 percent to 5 percent, a significant improvement.

Listeriosis

This is an illness from a bacteria found in some foods. You should avoid soft cheese that is not pasteurized, uncooked meats, fish, eggs, and raw shellfish. This does not mean you cannot have a few pieces of sushi or luncheon meats on occasion. Just make certain you get these products from very reputable distributors. The chance of contracting listeriosis is low.

Toxoplasmosis

Toxoplasmosis is a parasite that has to live on the body of an animal, such as a rodent or cat, to survive. In addition, vegetables and undercooked meats can carry this germ. Most people associate changing the cat litter box with contracting toxoplasmosis. This is true, but anyone in the room with the cat litter box can get the infection because the germs float in the air.

There is usually no way to determine if you have or have had toxoplasmosis unless you have a positive blood test. One-third of the entire population has been exposed to this germ and has antibodies that protect the fetus from any serious problems if exposed again. The fetus can develop anemia, requiring a transfusion in the womb, but this is rare. I have transfused three fetuses in the womb for toxoplasmosis, and all three babies did well. It is very rare that the fetus will have serious problems after birth if exposed during the pregnancy.

If you find that your first exposure to toxoplasmosis occurred during the second or third trimester, you should see a high-risk obstetrician for an evaluation. If you have to work in the yard or with cat litter, wear gloves, wash your hands, and wear a mask.

 ## Group B Streptococcal (GBS)

Group B streptococcal disease is a bacterial infection that can occur in pregnant women, newborn babies, those with chronic illnesses, and the elderly. *GBS is the most common cause of life-threatening infection in newborns.* It is the most common cause of meningitis and blood-based infections (sepsis) in newborns, and newborn pneumonia is most often caused by GBS.

Mothers can carry GBS in the bowel, vagina, bladder, or throat. Nearly 25 percent of all pregnant women carry GBS in the vagina or rectum. It is very easy for the fetus to come in contact with the GBS bacteria before or during labor.

GBS risk factors include:

- Prior baby with GBS disease
- Urinary tract infection associated with GBS
- Fever during labor

○ Rupture of membranes 18 hours or more before labor

○ Ruptured membranes before 37 weeks

○ Premature labor

All pregnant women should be screened for GBS at 36 weeks' gestation. Antibiotics should be given to any women who screen positive or if results are not available at the time of delivery. Although 100 percent of GBS can never be totally prevented, treating pregnant women in this manner will eliminate over 99 percent of newborn risk for developing GBS.

CHAPTER 49

Rh Factor

Part of the normal blood work for pregnant women is testing for blood type and the Rh factor. Blood type can be an important factor in a healthy pregnancy. Rh-negative is the only one of the blood groups that can cause a problem for pregnant women.

An Rh-negative mother can make antibodies against Rh-positive blood cells, even against those of her own baby. This is called Rh sensitization. These antibodies can cross the placenta and attach to your baby's red blood cells. This can lead to complications for the baby, including a low blood count (anemia), jaundice, and congestive heart failure.

If your blood work shows that you are Rh-negative, you will be tested for Rh antibody titers (anti-D). If you have not been sensitized, you will usually be given a drug called Rhogam. This is a special blood product that can prevent an Rh-negative mother's antibodies from being able to react to Rh-positive cells.

Rhogam is given to all Rh-negative women whose baby might be Rh-positive. The baby may be positive if the father is Rh-positive. If both parents are Rh-negative, they can only have a baby that is Rh-negative. Rhogam is given at times during the pregnancy when there is some likelihood of Rh-positive fetal blood getting into the mother's bloodstream.

Instances when a Rhogam injection might be necessary include:

- o   Amniocentesis or CVS
- o   Miscarriage
- o   After delivery

Because there is a risk of a placental tear during the third trimester, Rhogam is often administered after the 28th week of pregnancy. If you are Rh-negative, it may be necessary for a high-risk obstetrician to monitor you throughout your pregnancy.

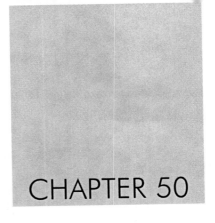

CHAPTER 50

Premature Labor and Delivery

Nearly 11 percent of all babies born in the United States are born prematurely, which totals a little less than 500,000 preterm births a year. Certainly, feelings of disappointment, fear, and even anger are natural and understandable for parents entering the world of the neonatal intensive care unit (NICU). The great news for new parents is that outcomes for these little babies have dramatically improved over the past 10–20 years.

The danger zone for delivering a preterm baby is from 23 to 26 weeks, and they are called micro-preemies. These very small babies are between 1 and 2½ pounds and have much higher risks for not surviving, as well as for brain damage, heart disease, infections, and other short- and long-term illnesses.

Babies born between 27 and 33 weeks do much better at being able to survive and get through common problems that affect premature babies. Those babies born between 34 and 37 weeks usually do well and have a very low risk of developing serious problems.

 ## The risk factors for premature delivery include:

- o Nothing at all! Over half of all babies born prematurely have no risk factors found in the mother.

- o A history of one previous preterm birth puts the current pregnancy at about a 20 percent risk for another preterm delivery.

- A history of two prior preterm births puts the current pregnancy at a risk of 50 percent for preterm birth.
- Smoking is a risk factor.
- Alcohol and drug use are risk factors.
- Heavy physical activity and long periods of standing are risk factors.
- An incompetent cervix (see chapter 36) is a risk factor, but placement of a stitch (cerclage) at about 12 weeks' gestation can reduce the risk factor.
- Chronic medical illnesses, such as high blood pressure, diabetes, and placenta previa (see chapter 52), are risk factors.
- Periodic vaginal bleeding from the uterus during the pregnancy is a risk factor.
- (Multiples)
- Twins: 25 percent are premature.
- Triplets: 70–80 percent are premature.
- Quads and more: 100 percent are premature.
- Teen mothers under 17 years old: 25–30 percent are preterm.
- Sexually transmitted diseases with active infections are risk factors.
- Too little or too much weight gain in the mother is a risk factor.
- Morbid obesity (mother's BMI >33 or weighing more than 250 pounds) increases the risk of a premature delivery.
- Dehydration is associated with uterine contractions. Drink at least eight glasses of water a day.

o Dental problems can occur during your pregnancy, due to hormone changes that make your gums bleed and more susceptible to infection. Infection in your mouth can cause bacteria to pass into your bloodstream, increasing your risk for complications, including preterm labor and possible early delivery.

What are the signs of premature labor?

o Repeated cramping in the lower belly

o Change or increase in vaginal discharge, which may include blood

o Thinning or shortening of your cervix, as seen by ultrasound, to less than 2.2 centimeters in length

o Cramps that keep getting stronger

If you experience any of the above symptoms, you likely will have a *fetal fibronectin test*. This test involves taking a Q-tip and placing it in the back of the vagina to test the vaginal secretions. If the fetal fibronectin (fFN) protein is present, you have a higher risk for premature birth. A positive fFN means there is a 50/50 chance of a delivery within three to four weeks. A negative test is good news for two weeks; there is only a 1–2 percent chance of delivery. Patients who have a negative test will likely be tested every two weeks until 34 weeks' gestation.

What can the doctor do to help my baby before delivery?

Your doctor may give you one or two shots of steroids before you deliver to help your baby have fewer problems with breathing once in the NICU. If you are carrying twins or more, your doctor may put you on bed rest early (28 weeks) and give you steroid shots should your water bag rupture early or if you need a rapid premature delivery.

❓ Are there medications for premature labor?

Yes, there are many drugs that have been tested and used for many years, but none have been shown to prolong the pregnancy for a long period of time. Our main goal in using drugs to stop your contractions is to allow time (24–48 hours) for the steroids that benefit the baby's lungs to take effect. Morphine, magnesium sulfate, Terbutaline, and Procardia are a few of the drugs that have been used to try to stop contractions.

Use of Terbutaline through continuous infusion has shown the most success at prolonging the pregnancy over other available methods. This treatment is administered at home and is used in conjunction with home uterine activity monitoring. I have used the Terbutaline pump many times over the years to prolong pregnancies of women with shortened cervixes and frequent contractions, extending their pregnancies from many days to weeks before delivery.

❓ Can a woman contract and not be in labor?

Yes, this is very common. Labor is happening when regular contractions are accompanied with a change in a woman's cervix. Frequent contractions with a negative fFN test probably mean that you are just dehydrated. Taking fluids by mouth or with the use of an intravenous line will often stop these contractions.

❓ Should a woman get a tubal ligation at delivery if she just delivered a preterm baby?

Most ob/gyn doctors do not advise a woman to do a procedure to end her ability to reproduce until at least six weeks after delivery, due to the unknown prognosis of the newborn.

❓ Do girls do better than boys if born prematurely?

The answer is yes, girls do a little better than boys, probably because of the presence of a different hormone mix in girls. All mammals in the animal kingdom favor females if born early, as the female allows the reproduction of the species to continue. You know, men are cheap, a dime a dozen. But women are the key for mankind surviving.

☉❓ What can you do to decrease your risk for preterm birth?

- Eat well, and do not gain more than you should (see chapter 13).

- Do not smoke.

- Do not use un-prescribed drugs.

- Get seven hours or more of sleep nightly.

- Let your doctor know if you feel contractions.

- If you have delivered a preterm baby before, see a high-risk obstetrician to discuss whether there are additional things you can do to reduce the risk of this happening again.

 ## Home Uterine Activity Monitoring

Using home uterine monitoring, with or without medication for reducing contractions, has been used and advocated for over 20 years for women at great risk for preterm birth or women currently being treated for preterm labor. Your doctor will discuss this service with you if you are brought to the hospital for preterm labor.

 ## Use of Progesterone to Decrease the Chance of Preterm Birth

For the past several years, researchers have been looking at the use of progesterone to reduce the chance of preterm birth in women with risk factors that move them into a high-risk category for an early delivery. The studies have shown that the risk of recurrent preterm birth is two to three times lower in women receiving

17-alpha progesterone, either by injection or vaginal suppository. The best method for delivering progesterone weekly to women at high risk is still being evaluated.

Progesterone supplementation should be offered to women with a history of a prior preterm delivery. Treatment should be started at 16–20 weeks' gestation and stopped at 34 weeks. This treatment will continue to be evaluated for several years to come.

CHAPTER 51

Premature Rupture of Membranes (PROM)

Premature rupture of the membranes is defined as the breaking of the amnion (water bag) before labor begins, which happens in about 15 percent of all pregnancies. Premature rupture has an association with over 50 percent of babies born prematurely. A weakening of the membranes from infection along with uterine contractions is thought to be the most common cause of rupture of the membranes.

 ## The risk of PROM is increased with the following:

○ Vaginal bleeding anytime during the pregnancy

○ Smoking

○ A shortened cervix coupled with a positive fetal fibronectin (fFN) swab of the cervix (see chapter 50; a positive swab means an increased risk of preterm birth)

○ Incompetent cervix

○ Poor nutrition

If you are 34 weeks or beyond, most obstetricians will deliver you within one to two days. If the PROM occurs earlier than 34 weeks, a prolonged hospitalization may be required, watching for signs of infection. If the fluid around the baby remains adequate, many women can continue under close observation for days to weeks after the rupture.

If the PROM occurs before 23 weeks and infection is present, then inducing and delivering should be started to prevent possible maternal septic infection and even maternal death.

There can be great danger from infection for both the mother and unborn child if the mother is permitted to go home with a ruptured water bag. Extended hospitalization is recommended if the fetus is viable (23–36 weeks) with close observation daily.

Women who have ruptured their membranes early in the second to third trimester may hear about replacing the fluid artificially. This has been attempted for many years *with no long-term improvement in the baby's outcome.*

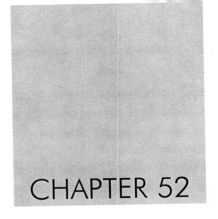

CHAPTER 52

Placenta Problems

The placenta is an unborn baby's support system. The blood vessels that attach from the placenta to the uterus provide an exchange of blood between the mother and her baby. This supplies the baby with oxygen and nutrients 24 hours a day for the entire pregnancy.

 ## Placenta Previa

Some pregnancies result in the placenta implanting low on the uterine wall, near the cervical opening. This occurs in about 1 in 200 pregnancies and can result in vaginal bleeding on occasion in any of the three trimesters. The most common sign of bleeding from a placenta previa is when no pain accompanies the bleeding. Often, a placenta seen very low on the uterine wall early in the first or second trimester will be pulled up and away from that area as the uterus gets larger. Your doctor will probably check for placental location periodically throughout the pregnancy.

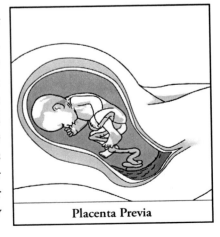

Placenta Previa

Depending on the location of the placenta, you may be asked to refrain from sexual intercourse until after delivery, as this activity under certain circumstances can lead to bleeding and even an early preterm birth. The location of the baby's head—and whether the placenta is in front of it—will determine whether you will be permitted to attempt a vaginal delivery or if a C-section will be performed.

You may also be asked to take additional iron so that you are not anemic at birth. This will reduce your risk of needing a blood transfusion.

 ## Placental Abruption

A placental abruption (separation) occurs when a portion of the placenta separates from the uterine wall. This can cause both vaginal bleeding and lower abdominal pain. Should you experience these symptoms, your doctor should be contacted so that you can be evaluated as soon as possible.

Treatment includes bed rest, intravenous hydration, medication to stop contractions, and delivery if necessary if the baby is near term.

The risk for an abruption can increase with:
- High blood pressure
- Smoking
- Women over 35 years old
- Women who have delivered more than four or five children
- Prior history of placenta previa
- Trauma to the mother's abdomen
- Use of illicit drugs (cocaine)
- Chronic disease (such as diabetes)

Complications include premature or emergency delivery, fetal growth problems, stillbirth, and brain damage to the unborn baby.

Placenta Accreta

A placenta accreta means that the placenta is deeply imbedded in the wall of the uterus and may not come off easily or at all following delivery of the baby.

If you have had a prior C-section, an earlier abruption in the current pregnancy, or a myomectomy (removal of fibroid tumors), then you are at a higher risk for a placenta accreta.

Having this complication could result in a hysterectomy at the time of your delivery.

 Subchorionic Bleed

A subchorionic bleed is a very common finding detected by ultrasound. This occurs when a small amount of the placenta lifts up off the uterine wall, resulting in blood accumulating beneath the membrane. This can result in an early pregnancy loss or a preterm delivery, depending on the location of the bleed and the amount of blood that has accumulated in that area. The majority of these subchorionic bleeds are short lived and the pregnancy usually continues with a normal outcome.

The risk factors for a subchorionic bleed include:

○ Placenta previa

○ Episodes of bleeding from the early first trimester

○ High blood pressure

○ Trauma to the belly

○ Cigarette smoking

Bed rest may be necessary for a period of time. Sex is usually not recommended during this time, as this can aggravate the bleed. Weekly antenatal testing is recommended starting at 34 weeks until term.

CHAPTER 53

Sexually Transmitted Diseases

Sexually transmitted diseases affect about one-third of all pregnant women yearly in the United States. An STD that remains undiagnosed or untreated during pregnancy can cause pregnancy complications and be harmful to your unborn baby.

 ## Herpes

Over 50 million people in the United States carry the herpes type 2 virus (the type affecting the sex organs of men and women). However, fewer than one in five people who have herpes type 2 viruses are aware that they are positive.

Classically, the initial outbreak of herpes type 2 is sometimes painful, causing itching and ulcer lesions on the penis or testicles in men and on the outer labia and in the vagina of women. In addition, viral symptoms that include muscle and joint aches, along with feeling tired, occur in some people. However, any person can get the virus without the sign of a lesion that hurts or causes itching. In addition, many men and women may get an initial outbreak and just think it is a pimple or hair caught under the skin.

If you want to know if you could be infected with herpes, ask your doctor for a blood test for herpes simplex virus (HSV) type 2. This test includes the antibodies type G (long-term exposure) and type M (recent initial or recurrent exposure). If you test negative, this doesn't mean you are 100 percent not infected. If you have recently been exposed, it may take up to six weeks for your body to build up enough antibodies to produce a positive result.

At this time, there is no vaccine or cure for herpes, but there are three antiviral drugs that are used to treat herpes infection. Acyclovir, famciclovir, and valacyclovir are all FDA pregnancy category B medications. All three drugs are approved for treatment of primary herpes, recurrent herpes, and daily treatment for suppression of recurrent herpes.

Primary genital herpes infection during pregnancy has a much higher risk of transmission than a recurrent infection. The risk of transmission to the baby from a primary outbreak at the time of delivery is about 30–60 percent with a vaginal birth. For women with recurrent lesions at the time of delivery, the rate of transmission is only 3 percent with a vaginal delivery. For women with a history of recurrent disease and no visible lesions at delivery, the transmission risk is only about 1 in 5,000. Cesarean delivery is not indicated with a history of herpes with no active genital lesions or prodromes. In addition, studies show women who receive suppressive therapy after 36 weeks of pregnancy are 75 percent less likely to have a recurrence, and the risk of needing a cesarean delivery is reduced by 40 percent.

If the newborn should get herpes type 2 infection, there are three categories of neonatal complications:

1. Localized infection of the skin, eyes, and mouth
2. Central nervous system disease, with or without skin lesions
3. Central whole-body infection affecting the brain (which can lead to lifelong complications or death)

The recommendation from the American College of Obstetricians and Gynecologists is that women with active lesions in the vaginal area (primary or recurrent) deliver their babies through C-section. In addition, if you feel that you are about to get a recurrent outbreak, but there are no lesions present, a C-section is again recommended. However, if you are HSV2 positive, have no active lesions, and feel symptom-free, you can proceed with a vaginal birth.

Though rare, herpes can still be passed through the birth canal, even with no active lesions present. If you know you are HSV2 positive and want to have a C-section even with no infection present, I suggest you talk with your ob/gyn early in the pregnancy about your feelings related to the mode of delivery. If you have never been tested for herpes, you can always have the blood test done, or if you find any type of lesion in the vaginal area, your ob/gyn can do a culture at any time.

 ## Human Papillomavirus (HPV)

The human papillomavirus virus (HPV) affects as much as 80 percent of the population. Most women find out they have the virus through an abnormal Pap smear or if they develop genital warts.

If you experience genital warts and are pregnant, you may find the growths developing faster and larger. This is due to the hormonal changes or lowered immune system associated with the pregnancy. While there is no cure for genital warts, it is possible to treat and remove them during pregnancy if they become problematic. Generally though, treatment is held off until after delivery.

Having HPV does not raise the risk of complications during the pregnancy but can be a problem during delivery. If HPV is active and you deliver vaginally, the lesions can tear as the baby passes through the birth canal. Although your doctor can sew the torn area, the pain may last longer and be slower in healing.

It is possible for you to pass the virus to your baby, but the chance of that happening is very low. If the baby does contract HPV, usually no treatment is necessary, as the baby will recover without any symptoms or complications. The majority of pregnant women with a history of HPV and warts go on to have healthy pregnancies and birthing experiences.

 ## Chlamydia

Chlamydia is the most frequently reported sexually transmitted bacterial disease in the United States, and about 10 percent of pregnant women are infected. Chlamydia is known as a "silent" disease because the majority of women have no symptoms. If you were to have symptoms, you might have an abnormal vaginal discharge or burning when urinating. If you test positive for chlamydia, it can be treated and cured with antibiotics. A single dose of Azthromycin or a week's worth of Doxycycline are the most common treatments.

If left untreated, this infection can lead to serious reproductive and other health problems. It can spread to the uterus or fallopian tubes and cause pelvic inflammatory disease (PID). PID can cause permanent damage to the fallopian tubes, uterus, and surrounding tissues, leading to infertility and ectopic pregnancy.

In pregnant women, an untreated infection can lead to a premature rupture of membranes and preterm delivery. *In addition, untreated women can pass the infection on to the baby during a vaginal delivery.* Infected babies can get infections in their eyes and respiratory tract that would require treatment with antibiotics.

 ## Gonorrhea

Gonorrhea is a common sexually transmitted bacterial infection that causes the same type of reproductive problems as chlamydia. Some women who are infected will experience vaginal discharge, burning with urination, and abdominal pain. Many women will not experience any symptoms of infection. If you are tested and do test positive, treatment with antibiotics will be necessary. This will prevent complications for you and the baby.

Pregnant women with an untreated infection are at an increased risk of miscarriage, premature rupture of membranes, and premature delivery. Babies born to women with an untreated gonorrhea infection frequently contract it during a vaginal delivery. It can affect the baby's eyes and joints. Life-threatening blood infections can also occur. If the baby does contract gonorrhea, treatment with antibiotics is needed. Babies usually receive medicated eye drops after birth as a preventative, in case infection went undetected in the mother.

HIV and AIDS

Human immunodeficiency virus (HIV) is an infection that can lead to AIDS (acquired immunodeficiency syndrome) and cause a breakdown of the body's immune system. HIV is caused by a retrovirus that can invade and destroy the cells that make up the immune system. This can result in a lowering of resistance to cancer and a variety of infections. *A pregnant woman has the ability to pass the disease on to the newborn.*

Often, the early symptoms of HIV infection are similar to early pregnancy and can include:

- o Fatigue
- o Unexplained weight loss
- o Skin infections
- o Recurrent upper-respiratory infections
- o Low-grade fevers
- o Swollen lymph nodes
- o Enlarged spleen
- o Diarrhea

- ○ Herpetic mouth sores
- ○ Night sweats

HIV risk can increase with drug abuse (especially injecting drugs), multiple sex partners, sexual relations with a bisexual male, and a current or past history of sexually transmitted diseases.

The pregnancy itself does not seem to be affected by mothers who are HIV positive. About 25 percent of babies born to untreated mothers develop the infection. However, active treatment of the mother significantly reduces the risk of transmission to the fetus/newborn.

Women with known HIV infection should take AZT from 14 weeks' gestation until delivery. The newborn should take AZT for the first six weeks of life.

 ## Trichomoniasis

This is a sexually transmitted disease that can affect the vagina, cervix, and urinary tract function. In pregnancy, trichomoniasis is associated with preterm birth as well as low birth weight. It can also cause the premature rupture of membranes. Some studies also suggest that pregnant women with this infection are twice as likely to have stillborn babies.

More than 8,000 pregnant women are infected every year with trichomoniasis. The infection can be difficult to diagnose because up to 60 percent of women have no symptoms. If symptoms are present, you may notice a yellow-green vaginal discharge. If you are experiencing any type of symptoms and are pregnant, it is important to notify your doctor, as testing for this disease is not routine.

It is very rare to pass the infection on to your baby during birth. If yours did contract trichomoniasis during the birthing process, the baby can be treated with antibiotics.

CHAPTER 54

Headaches

Headaches are very common during pregnancy, especially in the first and third trimesters. Most headaches experienced during pregnancy are tension headaches. Some women may experience migraine headaches for the first time in their lives in the beginning of their pregnancy. But on the whole, migraines happen less frequently.

During the first trimester, most headaches are caused by changes in hormone levels; most third-trimester headaches are caused by posture and tension from the extra weight you are carrying. Physicians generally recommend Tylenol (acetaminophen) for pain relief, which can be safely taken throughout your pregnancy. Non-steroidal anti-inflammatory drugs (NSAIDs), such as ibuprofen (Advil, Motrin, Aleve, for example), are generally *not recommended* during pregnancy, especially in the third trimester.

 Other steps you can take to help relieve or prevent headaches include:

○ Warm or cold compresses

○ Resting in a dark quiet room

○ Eating at regular intervals to keep your blood sugar from getting too low

○ Reducing stress

The majority of headaches that occur during pregnancy are completely harmless. At times, headaches can be a signal of a more serious problem.

 You need to call your physician if you experience the following symptoms with a headache:

- o Vision changes, numbness, or slurred speech
- o A stiff neck and a fever

If you have a headache in the third trimester with any of the above-mentioned symptoms, this could be a sign that you are developing preeclampsia and should not be ignored.

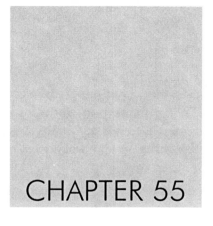

CHAPTER 55

Pain in Pregnancy

All women experience some sort of aches and pains in pregnancy, and this is to be expected. The good news is that the aches and pains you are feeling are most likely completely normal and nothing to worry about. The bad news is that you're feeling achy and in pain.

There are many different kinds of pain often described as shooting, sharp, burning, radiating, and aching. Below is a list of the most common aches and pains and what you can do to try to get some relief.

Back Pain

This type of pain is universal in pregnancy. This is why: a baby in that growing uterus causes you to push your stomach out for balance, placing incredible pressure on your lower back. The pressure is on your sciatic nerve, which goes down your legs from your pelvis, and only increases as you move through the pregnancy.

Steps to relieve the pressure and lessen nonstop back pain:

- ○ Take several breaks during your day to sit or lie down in a comfortable position.
- ○ Buy a pregnancy-support back brace. It can help

keep your posture closer to normal and reduce your backache. The extra support works for most women, but some women do not report any relief. You should wear it a few times per day when your back really hurts for an hour each time.

o Take Tylenol as needed. (Taking medications other than Tylenol can be safe during your pregnancy, but you must check with your doctor.)

o See a chiropractor or massage therapist. Make sure that they are certified in prenatal care.

o Avoid standing for long periods of time.

o Try not to lift heavy objects.

o When you have to lift an object, a person, or a pet, squat down, bending at the knees, and get back up using the muscles in your legs, not your back. Keep your back upright whenever you lift.

o Sleep on your side with your knees slightly bent. You can put a pillow between your knees or use a body pillow.

o Get your partner to give you a massage along your lower back.

o Use a heating pad on low.

o Take warm showers or baths.

o Apply alternating hot and cold compresses to your back.

This is an exercise you can try to reduce some of your back pain

Lie on your back on the carpet or a mat with a pillow under your head. Pull both legs up with your hands under your thighs and rock up and back for one to two minutes at a time, then rest for a minute and repeat for a total of 5–10 minutes. This puts your back and spine into proper position, allowing those muscles to

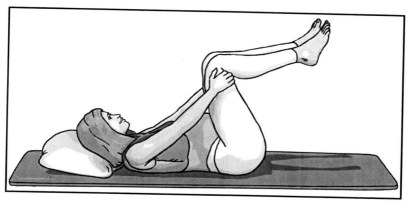

relax along your lower back. It will take that ache away or reduce it for a while. Do this exercise a few times each day.

Contact your healthcare provider if any backache is accompanied by any of the following symptoms:

- ○ Vaginal bleeding
- ○ Fever
- ○ Increased vaginal discharge
- ○ Burning while or after urinating
- ○ Uterine contractions (more frequently than every 10 minutes or lasting more than one hour)
- ○ Unusual pelvic pressure
- ○ Menstrual-type cramps

 ## Leg Pain

Leg pains or cramps may begin in your second trimester and get worse as your pregnancy progresses. Pain can be aggravated from the increasing pressure your growing uterus puts on blood vessels and nerves in your lower body that lead to your legs. While these pains and cramps can happen anytime of the day, they most frequently occur at night.

If the pain is persistent, you notice swelling or redness, or the area where it hurts is warm to the touch, you should contact your physician immediately. This could indicate that you have developed a blood clot, and immediate treatment would be necessary.

Tips for preventing or helping leg pain:
- Avoid standing for long periods of time.
- Do not cross your legs while sitting.
- Stretch the muscles in your legs several times a day.
- Take a warm bath.
- Sleep on your left side to improve circulation to your legs.
- Take a magnesium supplement.

 ## Varicose Veins

Varicose veins are very common in pregnancy, especially if this is not your first pregnancy. The excess volume of blood that you have in your circulatory system, combined with changes in the blood pressure exerted on your vascular system, promotes varicose veins. There is also a strong inherited (genetic) component to this problem; if your mother or grandmother had them, you might be more likely to have them too.

Minimizing the occurrence of varicose veins:
- Wear thigh-high support stockings from a surgical supply store.
- Avoid long periods of either standing or sitting.
- Keep your weight gain to a minimum (20–30 pounds while pregnant).
- Take a stool softener to minimize straining during bowel movements.
- Do not wear high heels.

○ Take a low-impact, 20-minute walk daily.

○ Take 500–1,000 mg of vitamin C daily.

 ## Pelvic Pain

At the end of the first trimester, women often begin to experience stretching of the round ligaments. These ligaments are attached on each side of the uterus and go down through your groin and attach to your vagina.

When the uterine muscle grows and begins to get heavier, the round ligaments are pulled, causing sharp pains. This pain usually happens on just one side. Using a heating pad on low and taking Tylenol is all that is usually needed to reduce the pain. It is rare that this type of pain would be from another cause, but if the pain is severe and persistent, you should be in contact with your healthcare provider.

 ## Braxton-Hicks Contractions

Braxton-Hicks contractions, also known as "practice contractions," can occur in the first and second trimesters; however, they are most common in the third trimester. These harmless contractions cause a tightening of the uterine muscle and may feel like a knot or hard ball in your lower abdomen. This tightening can last anywhere from 30 seconds to a few minutes and often happen sporadically, with no regular pattern. You may notice these contractions after sex, when your bladder is full, when the baby is active, and when you are dehydrated. Some women won't experience much discomfort when these contractions occur, while other women feel quite uncomfortable. Braxton-Hicks contractions should stop if you change positions, relax, and drink plenty of fluids.

 ## Carpal Tunnel Pain

This type of pain is very common in a majority of pregnant women. This pain originates in the wrists and goes down the fingers and up the arms. Numbness, tingling, aching, and burning pain can be present from early in the pregnancy, lasting until weeks following the delivery. There is a doubling of blood volume during your pregnancy. This extra blood and fluid in your veins and arteries makes the carpal tunnel, which is part of your wrist, become tight, causing this pressure and pain. Using a wrist support can help, as well as taking a natural diuretic (100 mg of vitamin B6, twice daily). Additionally, keep away from all added salt when you eat.

Occasionally, there are some women who have had injuries or certain medical problems that make the pain of being pregnant unbearable, requiring narcotics. As long as narcotics are taken only when absolutely necessary, the baby will not have any significant problems. However, if narcotics are taken till delivery, the baby will go through withdrawal for three to seven days after birth. If you are taking narcotic medications for any reason, make certain your doctor notifies pediatrics when the baby is born.

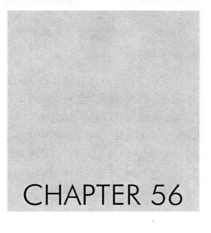

CHAPTER 56

Vaginal Discharge during Pregnancy

Most women have an increase in vaginal discharge throughout pregnancy, and this is normal. In the second and third trimesters, women often confuse increased vaginal discharge with ruptured membranes.

Ruptured membranes cause a watery and slightly yellow flow from the vagina. There are two or more cups of amniotic fluid in the second trimester and four or more cups in the third trimester. Again, amniotic fluid is fetal urine and usually continues to pour out if the membranes are ruptured. The fluid is continuously produced by the fetus, and if the mother thinks that her water bag has ruptured, she should contact her obstetrician and be seen right away.

Sometimes a woman can lose some of her own urine, which is mistaken for amniotic fluid, but your doctor will be able to determine the cause for a watery vaginal discharge.

In the last few weeks of the pregnancy, the mucus plug can be passed from the cervix through the vagina. It can be greenish yellow or bloody. This can mean that the cervix is thinning out and sometimes indicates that labor is going to start soon. However, passing this mucus can happen days to weeks before labor.

Thick mucus coupled with itching or burning can indicate

a vaginal infection. It can be treated with metronidazole (Flagyl, MetroGel). This drug is safe to take during the second and third trimesters. Yeast infections are also common and can be treated with over-the-counter creams. These meds are also safe to use during pregnancy. Vaginal and yeast infections can increase the risk for premature rupture of membranes as well as amniotic fluid infection if left untreated (see chapter 48).

 ## Six reasons to contact your doctor if you experience a vaginal discharge:

- ○ Foul-smelling discharge
- ○ Thick, curd-like discharge
- ○ Associated abdominal pain
- ○ Associated fever
- ○ Discharge changing to watery fluid
- ○ Associated tender abdomen

CHAPTER 57

Early Pregnancy Losses

The most common problem women have with a pregnancy is keeping it. In nature, depending on the mother's and father's ages, an early pregnancy loss (before week 12) occurs often. Many pregnancies end before the woman even knows she is pregnant. If you have had several children and never experienced an early loss, you are lucky.

Having an early pregnancy loss is just part of the miracle of having children. Most women who have had two children have had one miscarriage. However, having two or more early pregnancy losses can prompt your caregiver to run some tests to see if there are any associated problems.

? Is it common to have early pregnancy losses?

- Young women 15–25 years of age lose one in seven pregnancies in the first trimester.
- Women 25–35 years of age lose one in four pregnancies in the first trimester.
- Women 35–40 years of age lose one in three pregnancies in the first trimester.
- Women over 40 years old lose one in two-to-three pregnancies in the first trimester.

○ After the first trimester, the risk of pregnancy loss for women of all ages goes down to 2–3 percent for the remainder of the pregnancy.

Most couples would not believe it, but women getting pregnant have about a 10 percent chance of starting out with twins. Nature eliminates the twin pregnancies down to 1 in 80, which is the actual rate of twinning for mothers who give birth. So, losing one of two twins is very common and generally occurs early in the first trimester because of poor implantation or a birth defect. We did not know this until the last 20–30 years when close observation of pregnancies started with ultrasound. These early losses with twin gestations do not make the moms "high-risk" pregnant mothers, as it occurs so often.

❓ What could cause these early losses?

○ The most common reason for early losses is genetic, with 60 percent or more caused by an abnormal chromosome count (like Down syndrome or Trisomy16). In the case where two chromosomes are connected together, frequent early losses can occur. Your doctor will check the chromosomes of both you and your partner to see if you have a Robertsonian translocation (see chapter 28). This does not pose a problem for either you or your partner but can cause early losses in pregnancy.

○ Women with polycystic ovary syndrome have a higher risk of early losses.

○ Women with abnormalities of the uterus are at risk for having consecutive early losses. Multiple fibroids or a uterine septum that splits the uterus in half can be reasons for multiple losses and should be evaluated by your gynecologist. Surgery with a laparoscope can evaluate and correct these problems if your doctor feels that one of these contributed to your losses.

○ In addition, cervical incompetence (see chapter 36) can cause multiple losses, sometimes due to several D&Cs or cervical surgery.

○ Chronic infections should also be looked at as a possible cause.

○ Women over 30 years old start to have a higher risk of pregnancy loss, partly due to the age of the egg. By age 35, the early-loss rate is about 25–30 percent, and by age 40, there is a one in three risk. Once you reach 43 or older, every second pregnancy is lost, either naturally or from an increasingly long list of medical problems.

○ Women with antiphospholipid antibodies, thyroid antibodies, and inherited disorders like factor 5 Leiden and MTHFR (see chapter 32) all have a higher risk of pregnancy loss.

○ Over 50 percent of couples with recurrent early losses have no known cause. But more than 60 percent of these couples will go on to have a successful pregnancy.

Is it normal for a woman to blame herself for an early loss?

Women who have an early loss tend to attribute the loss to something they did, such as working, exercising hard, eating a certain food, vomiting, having a cold, feeling stressed emotionally, or any number of mundane events over the first couple of months of their pregnancies. This self-blame is simply not true.

What factors increase the risk of miscarriage?

○ Advanced maternal age (over 35)

○ Advanced paternal age (over 50)

- o Smoking
- o Use of street drugs
- o Morbid obesity
- o Diabetes
- o Chronic hypertension
- o Thyroid imbalance
- o Active sexually-transmitted diseases
- o Polycystic ovary syndrome
- o Chronic illness

❓ Will I need a D&C if I have an early loss?

Most women who have a very early loss, four to eight weeks, do not need a D&C (dilation and curettage). If you don't want to wait for a menstrual cycle, you can have a D&C, which is a short-stay procedure, only taking a few minutes to perform. However, if the loss occurs between nine and 14 weeks, a D&E (dilation and evacuation) of the uterus will likely need to be done. If you are much further along, 16 weeks or further, then you may have to go through a labor process and delivery.

❓ What can I do to reduce my risk of having an early loss?

- o Get your and your partner's blood tested for any chromosomal (balanced translocations) abnormalities.

- o Blood tests for anticardiolipin and lupus anticoagulant antibodies are also suggested. If these are positive, you may then need to be treated with low-dose aspirin (81 mg) and heparin during the next pregnancy. This test, if positive, may mean you have a risk of forming blood clots in the placenta.

○ Have a gynecologist evaluate you for abnormalities of the uterus or ovaries.

Mid-second trimester to term pregnancy losses are most often due to infection, premature rupture of membranes, placental dysfunction, and major organ system abnormalities in the fetus not seen earlier in the pregnancy.

Genetic testing can be done if you wish to determine if the loss occurred from the most common cause: a chromosomal abnormality. Over 99 percent of these chromosomal abnormalities happen in nature and do not run in families.

Because early pregnancy loss is a common part of nature, many couples postpone telling family and friends about the blessed event until the end of the third month. Just remember that more than half of all couples who have a pregnancy loss with the cause unfound do go on to have successful full-term pregnancies over 60 percent of the time.

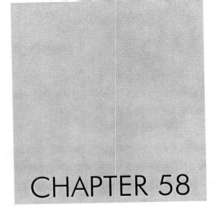

CHAPTER 58

Types of Pregnancy Loss

Below is a list of commonly used terms to describe a miscarriage or the loss of a pregnancy:

 ## Chemical Pregnancy

This is a loss so soon after conception that there is only an empty sac; no fetus actually develops.

 ## Ectopic Pregnancy

This occurs when a fertilized egg implants in your fallopian tube instead of your uterus. Rarely, a fertilized egg will implant on your ovary or on another organ in your abdomen. Women who have abnormalities of the fallopian tubes are at a higher risk of an ectopic pregnancy. Abnormal fallopian tubes can result from the following conditions:

o   Pelvic inflammatory disease

o   Scar tissue formation from a prior pelvic surgery

o   Endometriosis

o   A previous ectopic pregnancy

o   Sexually transmitted diseases

An ectopic pregnancy is usually diagnosed by a complaint of one-sided pain in the lower pelvis, an ultrasound evaluation in the first trimester, unexplained vaginal bleeding, or a slow-rising hCG level.

If caught early (less than 6 weeks), an ectopic pregnancy can usually be managed with the use of a drug called Methotrexate. This will cause the pregnancy to dissolve within the tube. If you are further along, you may need laparoscopic surgery to remove the pregnancy from the fallopian tube.

If an ectopic pregnancy is not caught early enough, your fallopian tube can burst, resulting in severe bleeding inside your abdomen. This can be very dangerous, and emergency surgery would be needed to remove the tube.

 ## Threatened Miscarriage

Cramps and/or vaginal bleeding can happen frequently in the early first trimester. Some women will continue on to eventually lose the pregnancy in the next few days or weeks. Doctors often call the bleeding and cramps that come along with a fetus that has a heartbeat, a threatened miscarriage. The majority of women who experience a threatened miscarriage go on to have a successful pregnancy and deliver at term.

 ## Inevitable Miscarriage

When cramps and bleeding progress to a point where the cervix opens internally, this is an inevitable pregnancy loss. This diagnosis can be made by exam or ultrasound scan. A woman with a diagnosis of inevitable miscarriage can wait for her period to begin or undergo a D&E (dilation and evacuation). I suggest that any woman with a loss or inevitable loss at eight weeks or further have a surgical D&E.

Incomplete/Complete Miscarriage

An incomplete miscarriage means that part of the pregnancy is coming through the cervix and out the vagina. Surgical assistance or the drug oxytocin can be used to completely clean out the uterine cavity. A complete miscarriage means that the woman has completely passed the pregnancy through the birth canal. She may need medication to make the uterus contract so that the bleeding will decrease.

Second- or Third-Trimester Loss

Women in the mid-second to third trimester who have been found to have a baby with no heartbeat need to be delivered. Labor needs to be induced with oxytocin or other medications to cause the uterus to contract so that the fetus can deliver vaginally. Pain medications, morphine pumps, or epidural anesthesia can be used for pain relief. *Emotional support and counseling should be part of all post-pregnancy management in these situations.*

CHAPTER 59

Dealing With a Pregnancy Loss

The loss of a pregnancy is always devastating to a woman and her partner, no matter how far along they are. You have not only suffered the loss of a pregnancy but also the loss of future hopes and dreams and your anticipated role as a parent. From the moment you found out you were pregnant, you started falling in love with this little person growing inside of you. You may have never met this baby before, but the pain of losing him or her is just as great as if you had. Only someone who has experienced the loss of a pregnancy can really relate to what you are feeling. The feelings of grief, anger, sorrow, and failure can be very strong.

While it is normal to mourn the loss of a pregnancy, it is also normal to start to feel better as time goes on. If you feel yourself gradually becoming more depressed over time, it would be best to seek out professional counseling to help you through this process.

If you are a man reading this, I must tell you that even if a pregnancy loss occurs in nature for no reason, women will often feel it necessary to blame themselves for the loss. It can be hard for us men to understand how deep these feelings go after a pregnancy loss. It may seem easy to say, "Don't worry, we'll just try again and everything will be fine." Certainly, that will probably be true, eventually. But in the first few weeks or months after a pregnancy loss, your partner is sure to be filled with a lot of emotion. While grief can bring a couple together, it can also drive them apart. It is not important that two people grieve the same way, but it is crucial that they are there to support each other during a very difficult time.

One normal feeling is to want to get pregnant again right away after a loss, but you should wait a few months to give the uterus time to cycle a few times before it can be ready to accept a new fertilized egg.

Dealing with another pregnancy after a loss is also often difficult, filled with doubt and concern that another loss will occur. Feeling anxious is normal, but the odds are very good that you will have a successful pregnancy, especially if you had only one prior loss. *Remember: pregnancy loss is very common and a normal part of reproduction.* It is usually not until after two losses that an investigation is begun to find out why these losses keep occurring. The good news is that there is usually a medical problem or condition that can be treated to achieve a successful pregnancy.

CHAPTER 60

Accidents and Trauma in Pregnancy

Experiencing any type of accident or trauma while pregnant can potentially present a serious situation. Falling is certainly the most common accident pregnant women have.

Once you hit the middle of the second trimester, looking down to see your feet and the ground can get pretty difficult. Going up and down stairs can also get harder as each week goes by.

If you suffer a fall and you are hurt, you should be seen by your doctor or go to the hospital to be checked out. You will be placed on a monitor to check the baby's heartbeat, and your placenta will be looked at by ultrasound to check for any separation from the uterine wall.

The good news is that the baby has a lot of cushion inside to avoid being hurt. It is also very unlikely that the pregnancy will be affected by a minor fall. It is still always better to be safe than sorry, so make sure you advise your doctor if you do take a tumble.

Any pregnant woman arriving in the emergency room after having been in a motor vehicle accident should not be permitted to leave without having a full evaluation followed by a period of extended rest and monitoring. One of the silent but deadly complications of an auto accident is the placenta coming loose from the wall of the uterus. If this goes undiscovered, both the mother and baby can bleed to death in the next several hours to a day.

I usually check basic blood work and do a test called the Kleihauer-Betke test. This test determines if there was a fetal-maternal exchange of blood. Any woman with an Rh-negative blood type should get a dose of Rhogam to protect her from sensitization.

A hospital stay of 12–24 hours is strongly suggested if the mother was in a serious auto accident—for both maternal and fetal monitoring. Over 50 percent of unborn babies that die related to trauma do so from injury to the placenta. Direct injury to the fetus from trauma occurs in less than 1 percent of all cases. X-rays, ultrasound, and MRI evaluations may be needed, posing no harm the fetus. It is often critical to have these radiological evaluations of the mother; avoiding them because of fear of radioactive exposures to the fetus is completely unwarranted.

After a complete workup and 12–24 hours of monitoring, the mother may go home but should have three to seven days of rest and should stay away from work and any physical activity. The pregnancy remains high-risk till delivery, and weekly ultrasound evaluation of the fetus should start at 34 weeks.

8
PART

THINGS TO CONSIDER BEFORE DELIVERY

CHAPTER 61

Getting Organized Before Delivery

 ## Planning a Natural Birth

For the past many years, our society in the United States has looked at admission to the hospital for pregnancy as no different from admission for an illness. *But pregnancy is not an illness.* In fact, the vast majority of pregnancies require little or no intervention. Only about 10 percent of pregnant women deliver prematurely, and another 5–10 percent of pregnant women have medical problems that can complicate the pregnancy. Of these, only some women will have a pregnancy-related problem requiring hospital care before, during, or after delivery.

That leaves 80 percent, or 4 million women yearly, who should be given the opportunity to experience a low-level, "hands off" birth with the help of their healthcare provider. If you are considered a low-risk patient and would be interested in having a non-interventional delivery, talk to your healthcare provider early in your pregnancy about a labor plan for you. Your doctor will be able to tell you what services are available for low-risk women in the hospital you will be delivering at.

Many hospitals now have updated labor and delivery suites that are much more comfortable and have a less hospital-like feel. Obstetricians and nurse-midwives may also perform deliveries at free-standing birthing centers, which have a more homelike feel. Some of these birthing centers are attached to the hospital or are in close proximity, if the baby should need special care.

You should attend childbirth classes and learn as much as you can about relaxation and natural pain-relief methods. Read as much as you can about having a natural childbirth. The more prepared you are, the more likely you will succeed.

I have been dealing with complicated pregnancies for the last 25 years. The best moments are when I can work with a couple to have a natural, non-interventional delivery in a room with some nice music and dim lights so that both Mom and Dad can participate in this miracle.

Every childbirth experience is different. One can have problems, while the next one can be uncomplicated. As long as the baby eventually drops down into the vagina and shows no signs of distress, the odds of having a successful natural vaginal delivery are 75–80 percent, which are pretty good odds.

If you do not have the opportunity to have a natural birthing experience, please do not be upset. I promise you that whatever route your baby takes to get here will be an extraordinary experience you will never forget.

 ## Increasing your chances for a non-interventional vaginal birth

If you are completely dilated and do not feel the urge to push, you should rest for a period of time in a sitting, squatting, or standing position depending on whether you have an epidural or not. This is also known as laboring-down. This resting period will allow for the baby's head to descend into the vagina. If the baby's heart rate remains stable, you can rest for 15 minutes to an hour. By not pushing before you are ready, you will reduce your risk of an assisted instrumental (forceps or vacuum) delivery and a possible C-section.

Organizing a Birth Plan

A birth plan helps keep everyone on the same page regarding your wants and desires once you go into labor. You and your partner should make a list of issues concerning your labor, delivery, and recovery period that you can review with your midwife or obstetrician before the last month of your pregnancy.

These issues may involve the following:

- When you should notify your obstetrical caregiver that you may be in labor
- Use of IV fluids
- Use of pain medications in early labor
- Use of an epidural for labor
- Use of oxytocin to augment labor, if necessary
- A coach or family member in the room at delivery and during the labor period
- Eating or drinking during labor
- Holding the baby following delivery
- Having an episiotomy
- Having Dad help with the delivery
- Cord blood banking (see chapter 62)
- Breast/bottle feeding
- Having the baby room with you or stay in the nursery
- Length of stay following delivery

Your provider likely has pre-registration forms that you can fill out and take to the hospital before your delivery. It is always best to do this beforehand. Filling out forms is probably the last thing you want to be doing while in labor. Many women will take the forms over to the hospital on the day they set up to tour labor and delivery to familiarize themselves with the lay of the land.

Your provider may also be able to give you a schedule of childbirth or new-parent classes at the hospital where you will be delivering. If not, give the hospital a call, and they will give you all that information.

To Doula or not to Doula?

More couples are utilizing the help of a doula these days before and after delivery. A doula is a specially trained woman who will act as your labor coach. She is usually a mother herself and will often meet with you several times before the delivery to work with you on the birth plan you will give to your midwife or physician.

A doula can act as a mediator between your healthcare provider and you and your partner. The doula does not perform the delivery but can assist your healthcare provider. Doulas give extra emotional support and confidence to the soon-to-be mom and dad. They will be there to support you in those first few days or weeks of being a new parent.

Before you hire a doula, set up a meeting with her to see if you feel comfortable with her. Doulas should not discourage or encourage any particular type of pain relief during labor, but support whatever you feel most comfortable with. She will help to educate you on what your options are for your labor and delivery. The hospital labor and delivery suite, as well as your healthcare provider, may be able to give you a list of names of recommended doulas in your community.

Finding a Pediatrician

If this is your first baby, it would be a good idea to choose a pediatrician before your baby arrives. You can ask your obstetrician to offer a recommendation, or you can ask friends who already have children if they have someone you might like.

You can then call a few pediatricians to set up an appointment and meet with them. They usually have certain days set aside for appointments to meet with parents to discuss their general philosophies on treatment and care. You may meet in a group of parents, but you will be able to ask any questions that concern you.

Some women like to choose a pediatrician that has privileges at the hospital where they want to deliver so that he or she can come evaluate the baby after it is born. If you find one that you like who does not have privileges at your hospital, you need not worry about the baby being evaluated. An attending pediatrician at the hospital will give your baby a complete examination to make sure all is well.

CHAPTER 62

Storing Umbilical Cord Blood

Stem cells represent a new area of medicine that will be used to help the outcome of many diseases in the future. The use of umbilical cord stem cells for treatment of leukemias and other childhood diseases has shown great promise over the past 15 years. This has resulted in 2–3 million couples spending several thousand dollars to store their baby's umbilical cord blood.

Everyone should know that private storage companies may not present fair and honest information about this service to the general public. For this reason, the major medical organizations in this country do not support the storage of umbilical cord blood in for-profit facilities for the low-risk couple, because the chance of needing it for their child is extremely low (1 in 20,000). Many states have free, public storage banks for umbilical cord blood for anyone to use. These are very high-quality facilities. However, if anyone's child from the public bank gets a cancer or chronic illness, then any cord blood sample in the center can be used, providing it is a match.

 ## Facts about Umbilical Stem Cell Storage

- The American Medical Association, the American Academy of Pediatrics, and the American College of Obstetrics and Gynecologists feel that storing umbilical blood is a reasonable procedure if you have a history in the family of childhood leukemias or other chronic childhood illnesses. However, if you do not, then it is not recommended as the chance of ever using this stored blood (stem cells) is extremely small.

○ Most types of childhood cancers that could benefit from these stem cells cannot use the umbilical cord blood that may have been stored from the affected child; they can use only stem cells from the cord blood of a sibling (brother or sister) or a donor. This is because the stem cells collected from the affected child could continue to promote cancer.

○ Only several hundred children to date have needed the stem cells stored from cord blood of well over 1 million specimens currently being stored. Only 1 in 10,000–100,000 stored cord blood specimens will be used to help save the life of one of these children. In addition, large blood banks can offer help to children from the thousands of anonymous specimens stored without charge in most major cities.

❓ How do I get counseling about the use of storing umbilical cord blood at my delivery?

Fair and unbiased counseling on this subject is very hard to find. Most doctors do not have a background in this new technology, only knowing what they've been told by the for-profit companies storing specimens from pregnant women.

❓ Is it true that these stored stem cells from my baby's umbilical cord can be used for older adults in the family for diseases?

No, but many for-profit companies will tell couples that adults in the family will soon be able to benefit from these stored umbilical cord cells. Cell laboratories may be able to learn techniques to grow the umbilical cord stem cells to an amount that is needed to benefit an adult for the treatment of chronic illnesses. However, to date, these stored stem cells can benefit only a person who is under 70–100 pounds.

What does it cost to store these umbilical cord blood cells?

The cost ranges from $2,500–$3,500 over the 17–19 years they will be stored. Usually that fee is paid up front.

Do you advise a couple to store umbilical cord blood?

I always counsel a couple regarding their chances of needing stored stem cells for their children. I recommend storing stem cells only if they have a child suffering with cancer or another chronic illness in their family.

I have been a cell biologist and geneticist for over 30 years and feel that stem cells will be used over the next 50–100 years in all areas of medicine to help treat and cure diseases and extend life. However, umbilical cord stem-cell storage has a limited use at this time. We are in the very early stages of this new and promising technology.

PART

9

PART

LABOR, DELIVERY AND POSTPARTUM

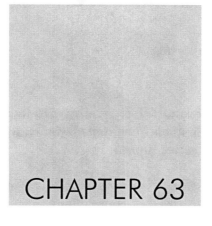

CHAPTER 63

Early Labor

The majority of women experience some of the early signs of labor weeks before their actual due date. Other women experience early signs of labor just a few hours before going into active labor. These signs help an expectant mother prepare her body for the upcoming delivery.

 Early Signs of Labor

Baby Dropping
This is also called *lightening*. As you get closer to your due date, you may feel the baby moving lower into your pelvic area.

Ripening of the Cervix
Your cervix will start to soften and thin out. This is called *effacing*. You will not know that it is happening, but it can be felt through a pelvic exam.

Bloody Show
During pregnancy, your cervical opening is blocked with a thick plug of mucus that keeps bacteria from getting into your uterus. The mucus plug may become dislodged when your cervix begins to efface.

Water Breaking

On occasion, the amniotic sac will start to leak or break before labor begins. Only about 15 percent of women actually break their water bag before active labor.

Contractions

You will start experiencing contractions that are stronger than Braxton-Hicks contractions. They will likely become more regular and intense.

Nesting Instinct

You may experience a sudden boost of energy, causing you to clean and organize in preparation for the baby.

 ## When to Call the Doctor

As you get closer to your delivery date, your doctor will talk to you about the signs of labor and when you should call. You will likely be told to call when your contractions are three to five minutes apart, or if you begin to leak fluid or start bleeding.

You should not worry that you will not get to the hospital in time. Just about everyone gets there in plenty of time. Make sure that you have your bag packed for the hospital in advance, just in case.

Do not be upset if you get to the hospital and are sent home. You will be kept only if you are regularly contracting, your cervix has made a change, and it has been confirmed that your water bag has broken, or if there are any signs of infection.

CHAPTER 64

Active Labor and Delivery

You have waited nine long months for this moment, and it has finally arrived. If this is your first baby, it is completely normal to feel some apprehension. It is not uncommon for me to hear a patient say, "I don't know if I can do this." I don't know if it helps to hear this or not, but I have never had a patient not be able to do it.

You can do everything possible to have the best and most uneventful pregnancy possible, but labor and delivery is always a toss-up as to whether it will go smoothly or not so smoothly. Try not to be disappointed if you had a birth plan and everything doesn't go exactly as you planned it would. The most important thing is that your baby arrives here safely and healthy.

 ## Admission to the Hospital for Labor

Once it has been confirmed that you are in fact in labor, you will be admitted to the hospital. Once admitted, you will be taken to your labor room and asked to change into a hospital gown. The initial evaluation will then be started, which includes taking a couple of tubes of blood and a urine specimen for evaluation.

You will then be placed on a monitor to determine how frequently you are contracting and to pick up the baby's heartbeat. You may be placed on IV fluids or be permitted to walk around in early labor without an IV in your arm. This depends on your hospital and doctor's policy on patients in labor. If you plan on having an epidural, you will need to be on IV fluids shortly after your admission. Patients are permitted to use the bathroom until they have a functioning epidural.

You can expect to be evaluated for cervical changes periodically during labor. This may be done by a nurse, your midwife, your ob/gyn, or an ob/gyn resident.

So, What's in the Delivery Room?

- There is a special bed that goes up and down and splits apart at the bottom so that you can put your feet and legs in special supports for the delivery.
- There is a blood pressure cuff.
- There is an oxygen outlet, in case it is necessary to give the baby (through you) a little extra oxygen. This is done if it looks like the baby is getting a little tired of those contractions and its heart rate starts to drop.
- There is a fetal heart rate monitor that looks like an EKG machine, which records your contractions and the baby's heart rate. There are little black belts that go around your waist with pressure and sound detectors built in.
- There is a newborn bassinet for your baby with all the bells and whistles: oxygen if it's necessary and bright lights to examine the baby.
- An IV pail will be next to your bed for IV fluids, in case you need them or are getting an epidural for labor.
- Last but not least, there is a nice chair for your partner and/or labor coach.

Fetal Monitoring

Today, continuous fetal heart rate tracing and contraction monitoring are the standard of care for all women in active labor across the United States.

When you are admitted for labor, you will be on the fetal monitor for at least a half hour and up to 45 minutes. At this point, if you want to get up and walk around a bit, you may do so if the baby's heart rate tracing appears normal. Once you are in active labor, you will remain on continuous monitoring, and if you need to get up, you will need to ask the nurse for assistance.

The rule of thumb is if it has been a normal pregnancy and the mother has come to the hospital in labor with a normal fetal heart rate tracing (heart rate 120–160 beats per minute), fewer than 5 in 100 babies will need a C-section for what we now call *non-reassuring fetal heart rate tracing*. This is what we used to call "fetal distress."

 Can I Eat and Drink during Labor?

Well, it is fine with me, but most ob/gyns, healthcare providers, and hospitals have rules that ice chips are all that will pass between your lips till the baby is out. This does not make sense because research has shown that labors are one to two hours shorter for women who are permitted to drink and have a "light" meal or snacks during labor. The thinking is that you could be at risk for choking on the food and drink if you needed to be put to sleep for a C-section. In fact, the risk of choking this way is less than 1 in 1 million.

 Positions for Labor

There are many effective positions you can try, but I wouldn't concentrate on any particular one until you find the one that is comfortable and effective for you! Positions like rocking, squatting, sitting, kneeling, lying on your side, or using a birthing ball may help you. You may find that a position that worked in early labor is no longer working as you approach delivery.

 ## The Three Stages of Labor

○ **Stage One**

This is the stage when a woman is regularly contracting every three to five minutes and the cervix is dilating. Active labor will continue to progress to more painful contractions as you continue to dilate. If the baby's head does not drop down into the pelvis, you will slow down or stop dilating. If your water bag has not broken during this stage and your doctor feels you are not progressing at a normal rate, you may have your water broken artificially. Some doctors will choose not to do this and begin administering Pitocin. Pitocin, a synthetic oxytocin, is often used to strengthen the contractions and help the baby move deeper into the pelvis. Your cervix must dilate to 10 cm in order to start pushing. Stage One of labor will usually last an average of 6–10 hours for a first pregnancy. A second pregnancy can be much faster.

○ **Stage Two**

This is the stage when your cervix is completely dilated and you begin pushing. The contractions are now very intense, and you will have a natural urge to push. You will likely feel a lot of pressure in your rectum. Do not worry or be embarrassed if you have a bowel movement while pushing. This happens often and is to be expected. The contractions will last 45–90 seconds with a two- to four-minute break in between. During each contraction, you will hold your breath

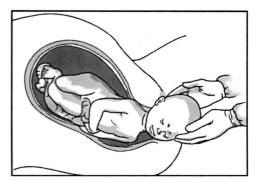

and push for a count of 10 seconds. You will take a breath and push again for another count of 10 seconds. You may be able to get three pushes out of one contraction. The baby's head will eventually crown, and the doctor will tell you to stop pushing so that they can position the baby for a final push that gets the head out. Once the head is out, the doctor will suction the baby's airway. The doctor will likely ask you to give one more little push to guide the baby's shoulders out. When the baby is out, the doctor will ask if your partner wants to cut the cord as it is being clamped. The entire process of the second stage can last from 20 minutes to two hours.

After the cord is cut, the baby will be cleaned off and handed back to you for some bonding time before heading over to the nursery. The baby will be weighed and undergo an initial evaluation at that time.

○ **Stage Three**

Your baby is delivered, and now it is time to get the placenta delivered. Your doctor will usually massage your lower abdomen, and the placenta should come out on its own. If the placenta does not come out with massage, a push or two from you should be all it takes to expel it. During this time, medication may be given to make your uterus contract stronger to reduce bleeding.

 Episiotomy at Delivery

An episiotomy is the cutting of the area between the vagina and rectum (perineum), allowing for an easier delivery of the baby's head when Mom is pushing during the second stage of labor.

Fewer episiotomies have been done over the past 10–20 years, with more obstetricians and midwives encouraging a longer stage of pushing. This allows the perineum to stretch more, thus reducing the need for an episiotomy.

There are two main reasons why an episiotomy is performed:

1. To get the baby out faster if the heart rate is dropping
2. To prevent serious lacerations to the mom when the head is coming out

In addition, if the baby's head is out, but the shoulders are difficult to get out, an episiotomy can be done to make it easier for the body to come out.

Make sure that you discuss the episiotomy with your practitioner before you go into labor; make it a part of your labor plan.

Are there any advantages to having an episiotomy?

In general, most obstetricians feel that it is better to have a controlled episiotomy than to allow the perineum to tear. This is because a torn perineum can result in bladder and rectal damage, as well as long-term chronic pain, lasting from months to years. In addition, an episiotomy allows for a tighter repair of the vagina, which can be of benefit during sexual intercourse.

 ## Forceps

Forceps have helped doctors for hundreds of years to deliver babies safely. Forceps are a safe and effective way to get the baby out if the baby is in distress or if the mother cannot push the baby out on her own. The doctor should be able to see the baby's head at the vaginal opening before forceps are used. The use of forceps can decrease the need for a C-section in some women. Don't be alarmed if you see red marks on the sides of your baby's head following delivery. This is to be expected, and they will fade in one to two weeks' time.

Vacuum Extraction

The vacuum extractor is a little plastic/rubber cup attached with tubing to a hand-held vacuum-pumping device. The cup is placed on the baby's scalp, and when a contraction starts, the hand pump is squeezed to create a safe amount of suction on the baby's scalp. As you push, the doctor tries to gently pull on the baby's head with the vacuum, easing the head under the pubic bone until delivery occurs. No more than three to five contractions are done with a vacuum. If the baby does not deliver, then your doctor may decide to have you rest for a bit or proceed with a C-section. Every delivery varies, but your doctor has much experience and will give you the best advice on what to do during this second stage of labor. The vacuum extractor can cause the back of the baby's head to have a bit of a cone shape. This usually goes away in a few days.

CHAPTER 65

Immediately After You Deliver

Every newborn is tested immediately following delivery to quickly evaluate its physical condition and determine if there is a need for extra medical care for the baby. This very first test is called the Apgar test.

 ## Apgar Test

The Apgar test is given to your baby at one minute after birth and again at five minutes after birth. Five factors are used to evaluate the baby's condition. Each factor is scored on a scale of 0 to 2, with 2 being the highest. The best possible score a baby can receive is a 10. A baby who scores a 7 or more is considered to be in good condition. Some babies will score below a 7 at the first test because they may need a little extra time adjusting to life in the outside world. At five minutes after birth, the Apgar score is recalculated. If the baby hasn't improved to 7 or greater, it may need some extra medical care and/or close supervision. This testing is a score for the baby's health in the first five minutes of life. It does not predict long-term outcome.

Please see table 65.1 to see the criteria used for calculating the baby's Apgar score.

Table 65.1: Apgar Scoring System

Test	0 Points	1 Point	2 Points
Muscle Tone	Absent	Arms and legs extended	Active movement with flexed arms and legs
Heart Rate	Absent	Below 100 bpm	Above 100 bpm
Response to Stimulation	No response	Facial grimace	Pulls away
Skin Color	Blue-gray/pale	Pink body and blue extremities	Completely pink
Breathing	Absent	Slow/irregular	Good /crying

 ## How You May Be Feeling

Women can feel a wide array of emotions following the birth of a baby. Some women will feel an immediate bond with their new baby along with feelings of joy and excitement, while others will feel detached, sad, and anxious. The sudden change in hormone levels following delivery is usually responsible for these not-so-happy feelings. These feelings will usually pass after getting some rest and a good meal.

Besides feeling exhausted from all the hard work you put into delivering your baby, you will likely experience some physical symptoms immediately afterward that are usually short-lived.

Physical symptoms you may experience following delivery include:

o Feeling light-headed

o Shaking and chills

o Stomach cramps from your uterus contracting back to its normal size

o Vaginal pain and bleeding

- ○ Nausea/vomiting
- ○ Unsteadiness and weakness as you try to stand up
- ○ Headache
- ○ Flu-like symptoms

CHAPTER 66

Managing Labor Pain

There are many ways that women deal with the pain of labor. Any woman will tell you that the pain of labor was worth it for the reward that changes your life forever! A woman can reduce her own pain in many ways during labor, including sitting, lying in a comfortable position, or walking.

 ## Epidural

The most common type of pain relief in the United States is the epidural. Nearly 60 percent of pregnant women having a vaginal delivery choose an epidural. An epidural often permits a woman to smile through some very painful contractions. In addition, the amount of medication can be increased or decreased, depending on how much is needed. Epidurals given early in active labor have not been shown to increase the rate of C-sections. You may need some help with your pushing if you have an epidural. This is because you may not feel your contractions as well.

 ## How is an epidural performed?

1. You will first need an IV to make sure you are well hydrated.
2. You will have a catheter placed in your bladder

because the epidural medication can suppress the urge to urinate.

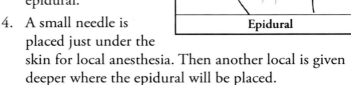

Epidural

3. Your back will be cleaned with an antiseptic solution, and the anesthesia specialist will push on your back to find the best place to put the epidural.

4. A small needle is placed just under the skin for local anesthesia. Then another local is given deeper where the epidural will be placed.

5. A longer, thin needle is then placed into the epidural location, and a catheter is positioned through the needle. The needle is then removed and the thin catheter is left in place, attached to a device next to you that will dispense the anesthetic medication through controllable, continuous infusion.

If the epidural is not giving you pain relief on both sides of your body, have your nurse call the anesthesia specialist. Often, an adjustment of the catheter will give you the pain relief you want.

Are there any complications from receiving an epidural?

Although rare, complications can occur:

- Some women might experience a headache following the procedure. If a headache does occur, it will usually subside within a few days.

○ An epidural can cause your blood pressure to drop. To decrease this risk, you will be given fluids intravenously before the drug is given.

○ After delivery, your back may be a bit sore. This is temporary and should not cause any long-term problems.

❔ Is there any reason that I would not be able to have an epidural?

Reasons that may prevent you from receiving an epidural include the following:

○ Orthopedic problems or previous back surgery where rods were placed into your back

○ Certain neurologic/autoimmune diseases that can affect nerves along your spine

○ A skin infection on your back

If you have any of the above-listed issues and want an epidural, ask your ob/gyn to consult with the anesthesia department prior to your delivery as to whether or not you will be permitted to have one.

❔ What about the use of pain medication?

Analgesic pain medications, such as Demerol, Morphine, and Pherergan, may be used either through an IV or injected into the muscle, but these medications go through to the baby and may cause newborn complications. For this reason, they are not the preferred method of choice for pain relief throughout labor.

❔ What else can I do if I do not want medications for labor, including an epidural?

You can look into childbirth education classes, such as Lamaze or the Bradley Method. You can also learn complementary alternative medicine (CAM) techniques for pain relief. These include:

- Acupuncture/Acupressure
- Massage
- Hypnotherapy
- Meditation
- Water birth

Obviously, you have to do some significant preparation if you are going to incorporate one of these techniques into your labor plan. Women in other countries today and many years ago used "mind over matter" methods to give birth without drugs. Childbirth is a natural, beautiful, happy, life-altering event that you do not want to miss because you're on "cloud nine" and out of it on drugs. Of course, the epidural is not like that, but you may want to try these other ways to get through labor.

If you have not studied and practiced Lamaze or other alternative methods before labor, I would recommend using conduction anesthesia like an epidural since this will have no effect on the baby. I do not recommend the use of narcotic pain relief during labor, as this will go directly to the fetus and can depress the baby.

Discuss all these options with your doctor long in advance of your due date.

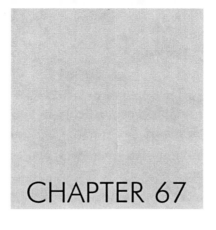

CHAPTER 67

Cesarean Delivery

Cesarean sections are done when labor is not going to result in a vaginal delivery, either because of problems with the baby or with the mother.

 There are also planned C-sections for many reasons that include:

- Multiple gestation
- Severe preeclampsia
- Complications of chronic illnesses
- A large fetus (greater than 4,500–5,000 grams)
- Severe growth restriction
- Patient's elective choice to have a C-section

 How is a C-section performed?

1. You will be wheeled into the operating room on your hospital bed, or you may walk in on your own.

2. You will be placed on an operating room table that looks like a small bed in the middle of the operating room and strapped in.

3. You may get spinal anesthesia for the C-section, which

takes just a few minutes to do and, like the epidural, gives you complete pain relief from your belly to your feet.

4. If the C-section is an emergency, you will most likely be put to sleep.

5. Once you are lying on the operating room table and the surgery is just about to begin, your partner will be brought in to sit next to you.

6. A surgical sheet will be placed to separate your upper body from your abdomen, which is considered a sterile area. For this reason, you and your partner will not be able to watch the surgery.

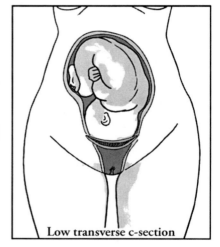

7. Usually a low incision is made just below your pubic hairline. The layers of skin and muscle are separated, and the surgeon then makes an incision in the uterus.

Low transverse c-section

8. The bag of water is broken, and the baby is lifted out of the uterus onto your belly. It is normal to feel a tugging or a pulling sensation and a lot of pressure as the baby is being delivered. But no pain. Often, we let Dad step onto the side of the OR table to cut the cord if he wants to do so.

9. The baby is handed to the nurses and cleaned off in the basinet. Because your arms are strapped down, you will not be able to hold the baby at that moment. The nurse

may bring the baby next to your cheek so that you can see and kiss your baby.

10. Meanwhile, the doctors are busy sewing your uterus and all of your body's other layers back together.

11. Some doctors prefer to close the incision on the skin with staples because they feel that the healing process can result in a thinner scar when no suture material is left under the skin. Dissolvable suture can also be used. This method is sometimes preferred by patients because there are no staples to be removed and the suture dissolves on its own. *You should discuss this prior to surgery with your doctor.*

12. You will then be moved to the recovery room for about an hour.

13. Figure you will be back in your room in about two to three hours.

 ## Higher Likelihood of Needing a C-section

One of the most common reasons a woman who is in active labor will need to undergo a C-section is if the baby's head does not descend or drop down into the deep pelvis, but remains high in the uterus. Reasons for this include size of the baby or position of the baby's head.

The use of Pitocin as an augmenting treatment is the only thing that can be tried to get the head to come down and allow labor to progress toward delivery. The use of Pitocin in this manner is not the same as an induction. The doctor cannot pull the baby's head down with the use of forceps or vacuum when the head remains too high in the uterus.

The following reasons do increase your risk of having a C-section after you go into labor:

o   Non-reassuring heart tracing or poor antenatal testing

- Type 2 diabetes
- Gestational diabetes
- Maternal obesity (morbid BMI>35)
- Multiple births (50 percent for twins; 100 percent for triplets)
- Breech position
- History of a prior C-section
- Low-lying placenta
- Maternal age over 40
- Growth restriction (small baby)
- High blood pressure on medication

Elective C-section

With the decrease in complications from undergoing a C-section, it has become more common for women to request an elective delivery by C-section. Women who are older and having their first baby, or are having a limited number of children, often want to discuss an elective C-section. The majority of women who choose this route of delivery want to avoid the possibility of vaginal tearing and stretching or future urinary and bladder complications. Some women choose an elective C-section to avoid the pain involved with a vaginal birth. Others may want to pick a specific date to have their baby.

If you are considering an elective C-section, I recommend that you discuss this with your obstetrician as early as the end of the first trimester.

If you are not planning on having any more children and would prefer not to use birth control any longer, you might be interested in a tubal ligation. Talk to your doctor about it beforehand if you want to combine the procedure with your C-section. Tubal ligation only takes a few minutes to perform, and the risks are extremely low.

CHAPTER 68

Induction of Labor

Inducing labor means bringing on contractions that will eventually result in labor, using a variety of techniques and drugs.

 ## Reasons for induction are for both the mother and the baby:

o **Maternal:** Preeclampsia, low amniotic fluid, diabetes, gestational diabetes, antiphospholipid syndrome, prior stillbirth, a history of heart disease or chronic illness, chronic hypertension, premature rupture of membranes, and post-dates (41 completed weeks)

o **Fetal:** Poor fetal growth, growth studies showing a large fetus, certain birth defects, and poor antenatal testing

Overall, labor is induced because it would be safer for the baby to be in the nursery, to lower the chance of a C-section with a big baby, or if the mother is ill and should no longer be pregnant.

 ## How is an induction done?

1. First, you will be examined by your doctor, and a decision will be made as to whether your cervix is favorable for labor, where you would then dilate

normally (1–2 cm/hour). A favorable cervix is one that is soft and ready to dilate. An unfavorable cervix is one that is still firm and may need assistance in being softened.

2.   A hormone substance called Cervadil is placed into the vagina for 8–12 hours. Some women will begin to have some contractions, while others will have few to none. The cervix can also be "ripened" with catheters, inflatable balloons, and a plant substance called laminaria, which is like a small, collapsed sponge that absorbs fluid and gets bigger. Made from a dried species of kelp, the laminaria stick or tent looks like a small cocktail straw. After 12 hours in the cervix, it will become as big as your finger and cause the cervix to dilate.

3.   The doctor will then start administering oxytocin. Mixed in a bag of IV fluid, the oxytocin will be increased slowly to help you contract. Eventually, the contractions will be every two to three minutes, and you should begin to dilate. If your contractions speed up, are too strong, or are happening too frequently, the oxytocin can be slowed or discontinued for 15–20 minutes and then restarted at a lower dose.

4.   Because an induction can be longer and more painful than the average labor, you should speak to your doctor about pain relief. An anesthesiologist will come to your room and go over everything with you.

Am I at a higher risk of having a C-section if I am being induced?

All women who are induced are at a higher risk of undergoing cesarean section. The chance of this occurring depends on the reason for induction and how dilated and effaced you are when you present for the induction. The overall odds of needing a C-section for delivery after an induction are about 30–40 percent.

❓ Can I ask my doctor to induce my labor a few weeks before my due date?

This is a common question asked by women who have had a difficult pregnancy or are just very uncomfortable and want the pregnancy to be over. The answer to this question is *no*.

Babies born 2–3 weeks before their due dates have an increased risk of being admitted to the neonatal intensive care unit (NICU) for respiratory problems and other premature delivery complications. The size of the baby does not matter. This is why all ob/gyn doctors are recommended to deliver a baby only after 38 completed weeks.

In general, an induction should be reserved for women with a medical reason for delivery or used electively after 40 completed weeks before becoming a post-date pregnancy.

CHAPTER 69

Complications of Labor

Although serious complications in labor and delivery are rare, problems can arise. *In most cases,* your healthcare provider can detect a problem and manage it appropriately before it becomes serious enough to put you or your baby at risk of a negative outcome.

 ## Malpresentation

Malpresentation or fetal malpresentation is where the baby is in a difficult position for the birthing process. The most common fetal malpresentation is the breech position. Rarely, a baby will present in the occiput posterior position (face up) or transverse position (sideways).

Breech Presentation

The majority of babies do present in the vertex (head down position) prior to labor. About 4 percent will present in the breech position. Recent studies in the past five years have shown that even in the hands of the most experienced obstetricians, there is a three to five times greater risk of a baby in breech suffering neonatal complications if delivered by vaginal birth. It is for this reason that the majority of obstetricians prefer that women with a breech presentation be delivered by C-section.

If your baby is presenting feet down prior to labor, your

doctor will discuss a C-section with you. If you present to labor and delivery fully dilated with the baby in the breech presentation, you will most likely be delivered vaginally. A vaginal delivery does have some danger, but at this stage it is safer than doing a C-section because the baby has already engaged into the lower pelvis. Pulling the baby back up through the pelvis and uterus can be dangerous.

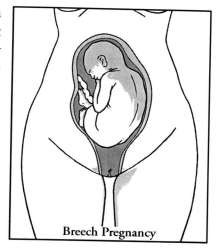

Breech Pregnancy

 ## Should I consider having my baby moved from the breech presentation to head first by my doctor with an external version?

This procedure does have risks, but overall the risk is low. The success rate of being able to turn the baby around is 50–70 percent, depending on the experience of the doctor, size of the baby, amount of amniotic fluid, and the position of the baby. During an external cephalic version, the baby can go into distress requiring a C-section.

Meconium

When a woman is in active labor and naturally or artificially has her membranes ruptured, the fluid is usually light yellow in color. If there is a brown tinge to the fluid, that means the baby passed stool in the womb. This can be dangerous if the baby shows signs of distress and swallows the bowel movement. This can cause respiratory problems, which usually can be treated after birth. The rate of C-section increases when meconium is present in the womb.

Shoulder Dystocia

This occurs when the baby's head is delivered but the shoulders are too wide to be removed and are stuck behind the mother's pubic bone or the opening to the birth canal. Your obstetrician will try many different maneuvers to help get the baby delivered. If these do not work, then the baby's clavicle bone (shoulder) will have to be broken to allow for delivery of the body. Poorly controlled diabetes, a family history of large babies, or the use of forceps to deliver the head can all increase the risk of shoulder dystocia. Usually, the mother and baby do well and do not have any permanent damage.

 ## Uterine Rupture

A rupture of the lower area of the uterine muscle can occur in women who have had a prior classical (up and down) uterine scar, multiple C-sections, a myomectomy (removal of fibroids), or multiple gestations. In addition, use of oxytocin in a prolonged labor can contribute to uterine rupture. It can occur at home before labor and can be "silent," or unnoticed. It can also be associated with severe pain following the rupture.

While in the hospital, loss of detecting contractions on the monitor and inability to hear the fetal heartbeat or feel the fetal head by an exam can indicate rupture.

An immediate C-section is necessary, as massive blood loss and fetal distress is common.

 ## Umbilical Cord Prolapse

Umbilical cord prolapse is a complication that occurs prior to or during delivery of the baby. The umbilical cord will drop down, through the open cervix, into the vagina ahead of the baby.

It is a rare event occurring from the following:

- ○ Premature rupture of membranes, especially if the fetus is in the breech presentation, may cause umbilical cord prolapse.

○ Artificially having your bag of water (amniotic sac) ruptured in the hospital with the baby's head not well engaged into the pelvis may cause umbilical cord prolapse. The cord can move down in front of the head and out the vagina.

Should you prematurely rupture at home and you feel the cord coming out your vagina, you should call 911 immediately. While waiting, lie down on your back with one or two pillows under your rear end. This will elevate your pelvis so that no pressure will be put against the cord. This is critical for the baby's oxygen supply. A cesarean section will be performed once you reach the hospital.

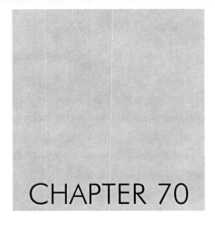

CHAPTER 70

Instructions If You Have to Deliver the Baby Yourself

If you are certain you are going to deliver immediately and know that you do not have time to make it to the hospital, here's what you need to do:

1. Do not panic—women have been delivering their own babies since the beginning of time.

2. Call 911 and let them know what's happening and where you are.

3. Try to get somebody to be with you if you are alone.

4. Do not push, but rather, pant to avoid tearing your cervix.

5. Quickly wash your hands and vaginal area with soap and water.

6. Get one or two large bowls and a few clean hand and bath towels.

7. Lie down on the bed or floor, with a folded bath towel beneath you to absorb the fluid and blood as the baby delivers.

8. If you feel like you are having a bowel movement, that is the baby's head coming down the birth canal and under your pelvic bone, putting pressure on your

rectum. Now you may actually have a bowel movement before the baby delivers. If you do, just try to clean it up the best you can.

9. If you feel the head coming out, gently put a little counter pressure against it, as if you are trying to push it back inside. That way, you are less likely to tear the perineum and vagina at the moment of delivery. As you apply this pressure in the middle of the baby's head, bear down, and gently push the baby out. Prop yourself up on a couple of pillows so that you can see what you are doing.

10. Once the head is out, use both hands to grasp the baby's head on each side and pull down gently as you push to deliver the shoulder. Once the first shoulder is delivered, gently pull the baby by the head and the free shoulder to the opposite side, allowing the other shoulder to deliver. The baby will then quickly slide out into your hands. Have a towel or two ready to lay the baby on, or bring the baby up onto your stomach.

11. Remember, the baby is covered with blood, fluid, and mucus—and is very slippery. Hold the baby firmly so that he or she doesn't go flying out of your arms and away from you.

12. Briefly turn the baby over and give a gentle couple of pats on the back, in case there is anything in the mouth preventing the baby from beginning to breathe.

13. If the baby doesn't cry or doesn't seem to be breathing well, you should take a towel and rub both sides of the body as well as the face and head. This will get the baby angry and cause him or her to fight back and cry and breathe.

14. When the paramedics arrive, they can help you with the

placenta, which may just deliver itself while you're lying there.

Good Luck! And don't forget that if this happens to you, your story will be told for decades to come among your family, friends, and neighbors.

CHAPTER 71

Vaginal Birth after Cesarean Section

VBAC (vaginal birth after cesarean) is the term used to describe attempting a vaginal delivery following a prior delivery by C-section. Having had one prior C-section, a woman may wish to attempt a vaginal birth for her next pregnancy. There is a 70 percent chance of a successful vaginal delivery in a future pregnancy if the prior C-section was not done for a large baby.

 ## The following are reasons that a VBAC could be considered:

○ The previous C-section was in response to a non-reassuring fetal heart rate.

○ The previous baby was in the vertex position, but face up, resulting in a C-section.

○ You had a successful vaginal birth prior to your C-section.

○ Your fetus is vertex and appears to be of normal size.

VBACs should *not* be done using an induction of labor by any means. This should be a natural labor only. If you are still undelivered and there appears to be a reason to get the baby out because of low amniotic fluid (oligohydramnios), growth restriction (small baby), or poor antenatal fetal testing, then a repeat C-section should be done. Inducing a labor after a prior C-section significantly raises the risk of uterine rupture, maternal bleeding, and danger to the life of the fetus.

 ## VBACs should usually be avoided if:

○ You have an unknown type of uterine scar.

○ You have a vertical (classical) uterine scar.

○ Prior uterine surgery has been performed (removal of a fibroid).

○ You have a multiple gestation.

○ The baby is in breech position.

 ## The advantages of a successful VBAC include:

○ Lower chance the mother will need a blood transfusion

○ Lower risk of infection

○ Less pain relief required following delivery

 ## VBAC complications include the following:

○ There may be an unsuccessful trial of labor, resulting in a repeat C-section.

○ A failed VBAC with repeat C-section can result in a higher risk of infection.

○ There may be a rupture of the lower uterus, resulting in an emergency C-section with risks to both the fetus and mother. This happens in only 1 percent or fewer of women.

You should discuss the pros and cons of attempting to have a VBAC with your doctor early in your pregnancy.

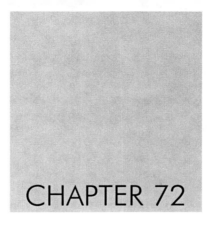

CHAPTER 72

Recovery after a Vaginal Delivery

Most women who have a vaginal delivery go home in 48 hours. Some women prefer to go home the following day. As long as you don't have a fever, your physician shouldn't have a problem discharging you then.

The recovery after a vaginal delivery is usually uneventful. Every woman heals in her own time, so don't get distressed if you know someone who seems to have gotten right back into the swing of things the moment they got home from the hospital.

 ## Pain Management

Pain is usually managed with acetaminophen (Tylenol) and ibuprofen (Advil) for a few days, if needed at all. An ice pack covered in a towel to avoid ice burn can be used to reduce pain and swelling.

 ## Vaginal Bleeding

Vaginal bleeding is very common following delivery and can be like a heavy period. Abdominal cramps are also very common. Do not be alarmed if you see some blood clots, as this is just a result of your uterus contracting and shrinking back down to its normal size. This is especially common in women who are breastfeeding or pumping their breast milk. If you experience excessive bleeding for more than a few days, contact your physician. Vaginal lochia (blood-tinged vaginal discharge) is common and normal for several weeks following delivery.

 ## Feeling Tired

Feeling very tired is not unusual after delivery, as women can be a little anemic. Anemia can contribute to that feeling of exhaustion. If your tiredness is interfering with your normal routine, it might be a good idea to go have your blood drawn to see if you are in fact anemic. If you are, your physician will likely start you on iron supplements.

 ## Bladder and Bowel Problems

After delivery, it can be difficult to completely empty your bladder because its controlling smooth muscle has been stretched along with everything else. This is the most common post-delivery complication, and you should be in touch with your doctor if you have an urgency to urinate, pain with urination, or tenderness over the bladder with a low-grade fever. Your doctor will check a sterile sample of urine to confirm an infection before treating you with an antibiotic. Leaking urine and not being able to control your bowels is very common. The nerves and muscles in the urethra and rectum get stretched from the baby passing through the birth canal. These problems should resolve themselves in 4–8 weeks following delivery. Numbness and pain in these areas is also very common.

Many women have some concern over the first bowel movement after a vaginal delivery. Some women will be constipated following birth and fear straining to move their bowels, especially if they have had an episiotomy. Use of a stool softener is recommended for the first one to two weeks following delivery. Do not worry that you will tear or that your stitches will break after a bowel movement. This would be a very rare event.

Episiotomy

If you had an episiotomy, you should take sitz baths in the hospital and continue at home for five to seven days. The hospital will usually give you a small plastic bowl that fits on your toilet to take home. The water should be mildly warm, and you should soak your perineum for 15–20 minutes, two to three times a day. Taking these baths will greatly help with the healing process. You should also wear loose clothing for a couple of weeks to keep your bottom from having any excess perspiration. These stitches are dissolvable and will not have to be removed.

 ## Hemorrhoids

If you were unfortunate to have hemorrhoids at your delivery, you will need some witch hazel pads, which will help with the swelling and discomfort. Sitz baths should also be taken two to three times daily.

 ## Sexual Intercourse

You should not have sexual intercourse until six weeks after your delivery, as it takes this long for your perineum to heal. It is best to wait until you have seen your doctor for your six-week check-up to make sure everything has healed properly.

Many women are nervous to resume sex for fear that it might be painful. I recommend women use a lubrication product the first few times, as there may be some soreness and discomfort. If you are breastfeeding, you will have higher prolactin levels along with lower estrogen levels. This will cause you to produce less lubrication during sex. A lubrication product will most likely be needed for a while. Sex might feel fine for you the first time you try. For others, it may take a few times before you feel like your old self again.

Kegel Exercises

Kegel exercises can be helpful after birth. These exercises help you regain bladder control, strengthen your pelvic floor muscles, and aid with perineal healing. To find the correct muscles, practice stopping the flow of urine when you urinate. Contract this muscle for 10 seconds and then relax. You should do this 10–20 times, three times a day.

 ## Breast Care

A few days after birth, your breasts will swell and become tender as your milk production begins. If you are breastfeeding, the best way to control breast problems is to keep your milk flowing. After nursing, you should rinse your breasts with clean water and let them air dry. Use of soap and scented cleaners is not recommended as this can cause the nipples to dry and crack. Special creams are available for cracked and dry nipples. You should not wear a bra that is too tight as this can cause a duct in your breast to become clogged. If you are not breastfeeding, you should wear a tight-fitting bra. Nipple stimulation should also be avoided until your milk has dried up. Ice packs can be applied for discomfort. If you experience any red lines or hard or lumpy areas on your breast, along with a low-grade fever, your doctor should be contacted. You may have a breast infection (mastitis) that can be treated with antibiotics.

 ## Exercise

Light exercise can be resumed when you feel ready, and regular exercise can begin four to six weeks following delivery.

 ## Driving

You should be able drive in a day or two after delivery. If you feel any pain when stepping on the brake, you should probably wait a few more days to recover.

Shifting Hormone Levels

You will most likely experience night sweats for a few weeks from the drop in estrogen after delivery. Hair loss is also common during this time.

CHAPTER 73

Recovery after a Cesarean Section

Recovering from a C-section is very much the same as recovering from abdominal surgery. Your recovery will be a bit longer and you will be more exhausted than if you had a vaginal birth. Most women typically spend three to four days in the hospital following a C-section.

There are two methods of closing the incision, one using removable staples and the other with dissolvable sutures. The staples are removed four to eight days after the surgery. Having the staples removed does not cause any pain. If your doctor used a dissolvable suture, it will not need to be removed but will dissolve under the skin within a couple of weeks.

 Recovery Tips:

○ Use pain medications for two to five days, such as acetaminophen, ibuprofen, and narcotics. I prefer to send the patient home with a small number of mild to moderate narcotic pills but always suggest using an anti-inflammatory instead, having the narcotic only as a back up if necessary.

○ Once you get home, you should have someone there to help you for the first few days.

- Avoid lifting heavy objects (kids, pets, groceries) for at least one week following your surgery.

- You may begin light exercise (walking, treadmill, etc.) 7–10 days after your C-section. Heavy exercise may begin six weeks following delivery.

- Do not go into a pool or the ocean before you see your obstetrician in five to six weeks following birth.

- Having sexual intercourse is not recommended until at least six weeks following your delivery.

- Skin creams that are used to make the scar fade should not be used until the scar is completely healed in one to two months.

 ## Reasons to call your doctor:

- Call your doctor if you have increasing pain or swelling around your incision.

- Call your doctor if you have a change in color around the incision, such as pink, red, or purple.

- Call your doctor if you have leaking fluid or blood from the incision. This can be part of the healing process, but you should make certain your doctor is aware.

- Call your doctor if you experience a temperature above 100.5°F.

Women who have C-sections will experience some vaginal bleeding, but not as much as from a vaginal delivery. Vaginal lochia (blood-tinged vaginal fluid) is also common after a C-section and will last for several weeks.

CHAPTER 74

Postpartum Depression

You just delivered a beautiful new baby and don't feel as happy as you thought you would. Feeling this way is actually quite normal—don't feel alone. Many women experience the "baby blues" in the days following delivery. If you have the baby blues, you may experience trouble sleeping, mood swings, no appetite, crying spells, restlessness, and a general sadness. These symptoms generally tend to get better over the next few weeks.

If these symptoms persist for longer than a month and you are having difficulty functioning in your everyday life, you may be experiencing a more severe type of depression called "postpartum depression."

Postpartum depression symptoms are similar to the baby blues but are generally more severe. You may not want to get out of bed in the morning, take care of the baby, or take care of yourself. If your sadness and hopelessness get severe enough, you might even have thoughts of harming your baby.

Some women do not feel able to share these feelings with their loved ones and continue to withdraw. Many hospitals now screen all moms for risk of postpartum depression so that proper support can be made available.

The most common risk factors that can contribute to depression following the baby's delivery include:

○ A prior personal history of anxiety and depression

○ A family history of depression

○ A complicated pregnancy or birth

○ Physical complications, including prolonged pain following delivery

○ A newborn with complications

○ Multiple gestation, causing increased exhaustion for the mother

○ A loss or lack of family support

If you feel you are in a depression that you just can't shake, it is important to reach out for help. Call your delivering doctor and let him or her know that you are having difficulty and need help. Your doctor can probably put you in touch with a mental health provider, if you don't already have one, and help make sure your partner and family understand what you are going through so that they can help you get yourself into a better state of mind. There are support groups online for moms with postpartum depression. It helps to talk with other women who are going through the same thing you are.

With the right medical help and support, you should make a full recovery and start enjoying life again, as well as that new baby of yours.

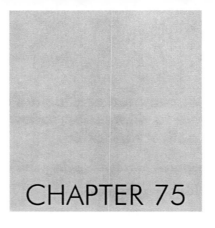

CHAPTER 75

Postpartum Hemorrhage

Postpartum hemorrhage is excessive bleeding following the birth of a baby. About 5 percent of women experience postpartum hemorrhage. Most cases occur within 24 hours following delivery, but it can occur later as well. Excessive and rapid blood loss can cause a severe drop in the mother's blood pressure and may lead to shock and death if not treated promptly.

 The primary causes of postpartum hemorrhage are:

○ Uterine relaxation or atony following delivery
○ Retained placenta, usually from a placenta accreta (embedded in the wall of the uterus).
○ Problems with clotting of blood
○ Inverted uterus (flipped inside out)

 The secondary causes of postpartum hemorrhage are:

○ Retained placenta or membranes
○ Infections
○ Inherited blood-clotting disorder

Factors that increase the risk of postpartum hemorrhage include:

o Prolonged labor

o Prior history of postpartum hemorrhage

o Induction of labor, especially if the Pitocin is used for more than 12–18 hours

o Preeclampsia

o Twins, triplets, or more

o Episiotomy

o Having a C-section

o Chorioamnionitis (infection)

o Rapid labor

o Problems with clotting

o Having had more than five children

What can be done to stop the bleeding?

o Pitocin (contracts the uterus)

o Methergine by shot (contracts the uterus)

o Prostaglandin (PG), F2 alpha (contracts the uterus)

o Massaging the uterus

o Packing the uterus

What happens if these things do not work?

Surgery would be performed to tie off arteries, and the last thing would be a hysterectomy.

CHAPTER 76

Thinking about Another Pregnancy

Choosing to have a second, third, or fourth child is a decision many parents might find themselves considering. Coming to a decision this time around might be more difficult than the first time. You have already gone through a pregnancy and delivery and have gotten a good taste of what being a parent is all about. Besides the emotional and financial aspect of adding to your family, there may be some additional things to think about before you embark on this amazing experience one more time.

 Things to Consider:

- If you are over 35 and thinking about adding to your family, it would probably be better to start sooner than later as conception becomes harder to achieve after the age of 35.

- It is always a good idea to space your pregnancies out a little, maybe 4–12 months after delivery before you try again. If you had a C-section, I would suggest at least six months before conceiving again. I am often asked how many C-sections are safe after having had one. The answer is that most studies state that three or four should be the maximum. Many C-sections put you in danger of risking a window or opening in the uterus prior to the next delivery. This can cause great danger to both you and your unborn child.

o   If you had medical or surgical problems in your prior pregnancies, talk with your ob/gyn about future pregnancies before conceiving.

You may be wondering about whether something that happened in the last pregnancy will happen again the next time. The general answer is probably not. Please see table 76.1 below for the chances of recurrence for a few common conditions.

Table 76.1: Common Conditions and their Chances of Recurrence

Down syndrome	1%
Preterm birth	15%–30%
High blood pressure	40%–60%
Placenta previa	10%
Preeclampsia	10%
Gestational diabetes	25%–40%
Postpartum bleeding	10%–20%

RESOURCE APPENDIX

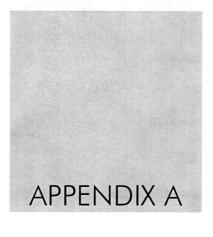

APPENDIX A

Important Contacts for Expectant Mothers

American Academy of Husband-Coached Childbirth
(800) 422-4784
www.bradleybirth.com

American College of Nurse-Midwives
(240) 485-1800
www.midwife.org

The American Academy of Pediatrics
(874) 434-4000
www.aap.org

American College of Obstetrics and Gynecology
www.acog.org

American Diabetes Association
(800) 342-2383
www.diabetes.org

Depression After Delivery
(800) 944-4773
www.depressionafterdelivery.com

Lamaze International
(800) 368-4404
www.lamaze.org

March of Dimes Birth Defects Foundation
(914) 428-7100
www.modimes.org

National Down Syndrome Society
(212) 460-9330
www.ndss.org

National Perinatal Information Center
(401) 274-0650
www.npic.org

Unite, Inc.
(888) 488-UNITE
www.unitegriefsupport.org

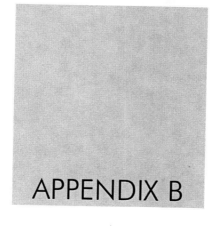

APPENDIX B

References

Immunizations during pregnancy. ACOG Committee Opinion No. 282. American College of Obstetricians and Gynecologists. *Obstet Gynecol* 2003;101: 207–12.

Obesity in pregnancy. ACOG Committee Opinion No. 315. American College of Obstetricians and Gynecologists. *Obstet Gynecol* 2005;106: 671–5.

Pain relief during pregnancy. ACOG Committee Opinion No. 295. American College of Obstetricians and Gynecology. *Obstet Gynecol* 2004;104: 213.

Perinatal risks associated with assisted reproductive technology. ACOG Committee Opinion No. 264. American College of Obstetricians and Gynecologists. *Obstet Gynecol* 2001;106: 1143–6.

Screening for fetal chromosomal abnormalities. ACOG Practice Bulletin No. 77. American College of Obstetricians and Gynecologists. *Obstet Gynecol* 2007;109: 217–27.

Umbilical cord blood banking. ACOG Committee Opinion No. 399. American College of Obstetricians and Gynecologists. *Obstet Gynecol* 2008;111: 475–7.

Vaginal birth after previous cesarean delivery. ACOG Practice Bulletin No. 54. American College of Obstetricians and Gynecologists. *Obstet Gynecol* 2004;104: 203–12.

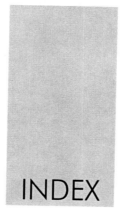

INDEX

American College of Obstetrics and
  Gynecology (ACOG), 9, 113,
  190–191, 224, 277
American Diabetes Association, 277
American Lung Association, 54
American Medical Association, 224
amniocentesis, 10, 15, 72, 81,
  82–87, 83*i*
amnion (water bag), 184. *See also*
  water bag
amniotic fluid. *See also*
  oligohydramnios; polyhydramnios
  levels of, 158–160, 203
  weight of, 44*t*
amniotic sac, 230, 255
anatomical abnormalities, 8
anatomy/anatomical ultrasound, 73,
  98, 105
anemia
  fetal, 172, 174, 176
  maternal, 1, 37, 42, 117, 120,
    164, 262. *See also* sickle cell
    anemia
anencephaly, 104, 105
anesthesia
  for cerclage procedure, 128
  conduction, 244
  during delivery, 139
  for delivery of second- and third-
    trimester losses, 212
  epidural. *See* epidural
  spinal, 139, 245
antenatal fetal evaluation, 90–91
antenatal testing, 7, 90–92
antibiotics, 120
antibodies
  anticardiolipin antibodies, 116,
    208
  antiphospholipid antibody
    syndrome, 116, 117, 207
  type G, 189
  type M, 190

anticonvulsant medication, 134
anti-epileptic drugs, 134
antiphospholipid antibody
  syndrome, 116, 117, 207
anti-thrombin III deficiency, 116
anxiety disorder, 142–143
Apgar test (baby), 238, 239*t*
appetite, 40, 141, 268
areola, darkening of, 19
aspirin
  adult, 53, 117, 118, 162, 208
  baby, 64, 65
assisted instrumental delivery, 220
assisted reproductive technology,
  8–10
asthma, 15, 91, 136–137, 170
autism, 107
auto accidents, 215–216
autosomal dominant disorders, 71–72
autosomal recessive disorders, 72
AZT, 194
Azthromycin, 192

B
baby aspirin, 64, 65
baby blues, 268–269
baby development, 29–33, 54. *See
  also specific developments*
baby dropping (lightening), 229
baby hair, myth about, 14
baby heartbeat, myth about, 14
baby movement. *See* movement, fetal
baby testing (Apgar), 238, 239*t*
baby weight. *See* birth weight
back brace, pregnancy-support,
  197–198
back pain, 197–198
backaches, 22, 61, 198–199
baths
  full baths, 15, 61, 170, 171, 198,
    200. *See also* hot tubs
  sitz baths, 131, 263

LaVergne, TN USA
19 December 2009
167559LV00003B/1/P